D1675998

 This book has been sponsored by
Sebapharma GmbH & Co., 5407 Boppard 1 - Bad Salzig

O. Braun-Falco H.C. Korting (Eds.)

Griesbach Conference

Skin Cleansing with Synthetic Detergents

Chemical, Ecological, and Clinical Aspects

With 89 Figures and 45 Tables

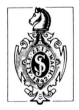

Springer-Verlag

Berlin Heidelberg New York
London Paris Tokyo
Hong Kong Barcelona
Budapest

Prof. Dr. med. Dr. h. c. mult. Otto Braun-Falco
PD Dr. med. Hans Christian Korting
Department of Dermatology
University of Munich
Frauenlobstrasse 9–11
D-8000 München 2, FRG

Title of the original German edition:
Hautreinigung mit Syndets.
© Springer-Verlag Berlin Heidelberg 1990

ISBN 3-540-55409-2 Springer-Verlag Berlin Heidelberg New York
ISBN 0-387-55409-2 Springer-Verlag New York Berlin Heidelberg

Library of Congress Cataloging-in-Publication Data
Griesbach-Konferenz Hautreinigung mit Syndets (1988) Skin cleansing with synthetic detergents : chemical, ecological, and clinical aspects / Griesbach Conference ; O. Braun-Falco, H.C. Korting, eds. p. cm.
Includes bibliographical references and index.
ISBN 3-540-55409-2 (Berlin : acid-free paper).
ISBN 0-387-55409-2 (New York : acid-free paper).
1. Detergents, Synthetic – Toxicology – Congresses. 2. Detergents, Synthetic – Environmental aspects – Congresses. 3. Skin – Care and hygiene – Congresses. I. Braun-Falco, Otto. II. Korting, Hans Christian. III. Title.
RA1242.D4G75 1988 92-13632

This work is subject to copyright. All rights are reserved, whether the whole or part of the material is concerned, specifically the rights of translation, reprinting, reuse of illustrations, recitation, broadcasting, reproduction on microfilm or in any other way, and storage in data banks. Duplication of this publication or parts thereof is permitted only under the provisions of the German Copyright Law of September 9, 1965, in its current version, and permission for use must always be obtained from Springer-Verlag. Violations are liable for prosecution under the German Copyright Law.

© Springer-Verlag Berlin Heidelberg 1992
Printed in Germany

The use of general descriptive names, registered names, trademarks, etc. in this publication does not imply, even in the absence of a specific statement, that such names are exempt from the relevant protective laws and regulations and therefore free for general use.
Product liability: The publishers cannot guarantee the accuracy of any information about dosage and application contained in this book. In every individual case the user must check such information by consulting the relevant literature.

Typesetting, printing and bookbinding: E. Kieser, 8902 Neusäss

27/3145-5 4 3 2 1 – Printed on acid-free paper

Preface

We do not know exactly when Man adopted the civilized habit of washing. However, personal cleansing (of a more or less regular kind) goes back thousands of years. Nowadays, the chief beneficiaries of these ablutional activities are the hands and face, which, being exposed, are more likely to collect dirt and grime. For a long time, the only cleansing agent (apart from plain water) was soap. Today, we have a choice: a new range of substances, the so-called synthetic detergents, have been developed. Unlike soap, these surfactants offer wide formula variability, and have, therefore, become increasingly important for skin cleansing.

With our growing perception, not only of the benefits, but also of the possible disadvantages, of skin cleansing agents, it was felt that the time had come for experts from the various disciplines involved in the manufacture and use of skin cleansers to take a critical look at what we know and where we stand. It was also suggested that this stock-taking should extend, equally, to the chemical, ecological, and clinical aspects of the subject. As a result, a meeting of 29 experts – mainly from the fields of chemistry, biology, pharmacy, and medicine – was convened at Griesbach, from 8–10 December, 1988. This monograph reflects the proceedings of the conference, including the results of the in-depth discussions of the subjects on the agenda. It is hoped that this book will help to spread our present, much enhanced, knowledge of skin cleansing.

Neither the conference itself nor the publication of its proceedings would have been possible without the generous support of Sebapharma GmbH & Co., Boppard. Our special thanks are due to Dr. med. Heinz Maurer.

Munich, May 1990 O. Braun-Falco · H. C. Korting

Acknowledgement

The editors acknowledge the support given by Sebapharma GmbH & Co., D-5407 Boppard 1 – Bad Salzig, in the publication of these Proceedings.

Contents

Preface

O. Braun-Falco and H. C. Korting V

The Use of Synthetic Detergents for Skin Cleansing
Historical Background 1

From Soap Avoidance to Skin Cleansing with
Synthetic Detergents – Moving into the Clinical Dimension
O. Braun-Falco 3

Skin Cleanser Chemistry
The Chemistry of Synthetic Detergents 9

Synthetic Detergents – Syndets – the Concept
K. Schumann 11

Soap – Chemical Constituents
G. Kolaczinski 15

Synthetic Cleansers – Chemical Constituents
W. Schneider 20

Composition of Commercial Synthetic Skin Cleansers
W. Schadenböck 27

The Use of Synthetic Detergents in Oral Hygiene Products –
Effects on the Gingiva
W. Weinert 35

Physiological and Pathophysiological Aspects
of the Use of Synthetic Detergents for Skin Cleansing
Skin pH 41

The Physics of pH and Surface pH Measurement
H. Galster 43

Determination of Skin Surface pH in Healthy Subjects
Methods and Results of Clinical Studies
M. Kober 53

Skin Surface pH in the Population at Large Measured Data
and Correlation with Other Parameters
K. Klein, H. Evers, and H. W. Voß 62

Skin Flora 73

Principles of Bacterial Ecology
W. Dott 75

Composition of the Skin Flora
A. A. Hartmann 83

Marchionini's Acid Mantle Concept and the Effect on the Skin
Resident Flora of Washing with Skin Cleansing Agents
of Different pH
H. C. Korting 87

In-Vitro Control of the Growth of Important Bacteria of the
Resident Skin Flora by Changes in pH
A. Lukacs 97

Skin Surface Structure 107

Structure of Human Skin, and Influence of Environmental Factors
Such as pH on the Growth of Keratinocytes –
Results of Cell Culture Experiments
R. Soehnchen 109

Skin Roughness – Measuring Methods and Dependence
on Washing Procedure
D. Vieluf 116

Skin Hydration (Transepidermal Water Loss) –
Measuring Methods and Dependence on Washing Procedure
H. Zienicke 130

Beneficial Effects of Synthetic Detergent Cleansers in Human Trials Under Simulated Use Conditions 141

Cleansing Action of Synthetic Detergents –
Methodology of Determination
K. Schrader 143

Clinical Assessment of Synthetic Detergent Cleansers
in Subjects with Problem Skin
F. Klaschka 154

Adjuvant Treatment with Synthetic Detergent Preparations
in Atopic Dermatitis
W. Lechner 160

The Use of Synthetic Skin Cleansers in Neonates and Infants
F. Braun, D. Lachmann, and H. Howanietz 164

Unwanted Effects of Synthetic Detergent Cleansers when Used in Normal or in Diseased Skin 171

Allergological Evaluation of Synthetic Skin Cleansers
J. Ring and R. Gollhausen 173

Factors Involved in the Irritancy Testing of
Synthetic Cleanser Constituents
R. Gollhausen 181

Quality Assurance and Environmental Aspects of Synthetic Detergent Skin Cleansers 191

Biopharmaceutical Aspects of Synthetic Detergent Skin Cleansers
K. Thoma 193

Quality Control of Synthetic Detergent Cleansers
K. Stanzl 203

Environmental Aspects of Synthetic Detergent Preparations
H. H. Rump 209

The Use of Synthetic Detergent Skin Cleansers 217

The Use of Synthetic Detergent Skin Cleansers –
The Cosmetic Chemists's View
H. P. Fiedler 219

The Use of Synthetic Detergent Skin Cleansers –
The Community Pharmacist's View
H. Führling 223

The Use of Synthetic Detergent Skin Cleansers –
The General Practitioner's View
B. König 225

The Use of Synthetic Detergent Skin Cleansers –
The Consultant Dermatologist's View
G. P. Heilgemeir 229

List of Contributors

Braun, F., Doz. Dr.
 Universitäts-Kinderklinik, Währinger Gürtel 18–20, A-1090 Wien, Austria
Braun-Falco, O., Prof. Dr. Dr. h. c. mult.
 Dermatologische Klinik und Poliklinik der Ludwig-Maximilians-Universität München, Frauenlobstrasse 9–11, W-8000 München 2, FRG
Dott, W., Prof. Dr.
 Fachgebiet Hygiene der Technischen Universität, Amrumer Strasse 32, 1000 Berlin 65, FRG
Fiedler, H. P., Dr.
 Lanzstrasse 4, W-6200 Wiesbaden, FRG
Führling, H., Dr.
 Josef-Simon-Strasse 4, W-8500 Nürnberg 50, FRG
Galster, H., Dr.
 Spessart-Strasse 15, W-6368 Bad Vilbel, FRG
Gollhausen, R., Dr.
 Dermatologische Klinik und Poliklinik der Ludwig-Maximilians-Universität München, Frauenlobstrasse 9–11, W-8000 München 2, FRG
Heilgemeir, G. P., Dr.
 Rathausplatz 8, W-8900 Augsburg, FRG
Hartmann, A. A., Prof. Dr.
 Dermatologische Klinik und Poliklinik der Bayerischen Maximilians-Universität Würzburg, Josef-Schneider-Strasse 2, W-8700 Würzburg, FRG
Klaschka, F., Prof. Dr.
 Hautklinik im Klinikum Steglitz der Freien Universität Berlin, Hindenburgdamm 30, 1000 Berlin 45, FRG
Klein, K., Prof. Dr.
 Institut für Naturwissenschaften und ihre Didaktik der Universität zu Köln, Gronewaldstrasse 2, W-5000 Köln 41, FRG

Kober, M., Dr.
　Dermatologische Klinik und Poliklinik der Ludwig-Maximilians-
　Universität München, Frauenlobstrasse 9–11, W-8000 München 2,
　FRG
Kolaczinski, G., Dr.
　Henkel KGaA, Postfach 11 00, W-4000 Düsseldorf 1, FRG
König, B., Prof. Dr.
　Prunkgasse 8, W-6500 Mainz-Finthen, FRG
Korting, H. C., Priv.-Doz. Dr.
　Dermatologische Klinik und Poliklinik der Ludwig-Maximilians-
　Universität München, Frauenlobstrasse 9–11, W-8000 München 2,
　FRG
Lechner, W., Prof. Dr.
　Universitäts-Hautklinik Würzburg, Josef-Schneider-Strasse 2,
　W-8700 Würzburg, FRG
Lukacs, A., Dr.
　Dermatologische Klinik und Poliklinik der Ludwig-Maximilians-
　Universität München, Frauenlobstrasse 9–11, W-8000 München 2,
　FRG
Ring, J., Prof. Dr. Dr.
　Dermatologische Klinik und Poliklinik der Ludwig-Maximilians-
　Universität München, Frauenlobstrasse 9–11, W-8000 München 2,
　FRG
Rump, H. H., Dr.
　Institut Fresenius, Im Maisel 14, W-6204 Taunusstein 4, FRG
Schadenböck, W., Dr.
　INCOS Beratungslabor Dr. W. Schadenböck,
　Galileo-Galilei-Strasse 10, W-6500 Mainz 42, FRG
Schneider, W., Dr.
　Henkel KGaA, Henkelstrasse 67,
　W-4000 Düseldorf-Holthausen, FRG
Schrader, K.
　Beratungslabor für die kosmetische und pharmazeutische Industrie,
　Max-Planck-Strasse 6, W-3450 Holzminden 1, FRG
Schumann, K., Dr.
　Henkel KGaA, Henkelstrasse 67,
　W-4000 Düsseldorf-Holthausen, FRG
Soehnchen, R., Dr.
　Dermatologische Klinik und Poliklinik der Ludwig-Maximilians-
　Universität München, Frauenlobstrasse 9–11, W-8000 München 2,
　FRG
Stanzl, K., Dr.
　Sebapharma GmbH u. Co., Binger Strasse 80,
　W-5407 Boppard-Bad Salzig 1, FRG

Thoma, K., Prof. Dr.
    Institut für pharmazeutische Technologie der Ludwig-Maximilians-
    Universität München, Sophienstrasse 10, W-8000 München 2, FRG
Vieluf, D., Dr.
    Dermatologische Klinik und Poliklinik der Ludwig-Maximilians-
    Universität München, Frauenlobstrasse 9–11, W-8000 München 2,
    FRG
Weinert, W., Dr.
    Blendax GmbH, Rheinallee 88, W-6500 Mainz 1, FRG
Zienicke, H., Dr.
    Dermatologische Klinik und Poliklinik der Ludwig-Maximilians-
    Universität München, Frauenlobstrasse 9–11, W-8000 München 2,
    FRG

The Use of Synthetic Detergents for Skin Cleansing

Historical Background

From Soap Avoidance to Skin Cleansing with Synthetic Detergents – Moving into the Clinical Dimension

O. Braun-Falco

Introduction

The earliest effective skin cleansing agent (apart from plain water) used by man was soap. The history of soap goes back some 5000 years. There are references to the use of soap in Sumerian clay tablets dating from ca. 2500 B.C. In those days, soap was made from vegetable oils and potash, producing what we would nowadays call a soft soap.

Unlikely though it may sound to some, the ancient Gauls and the Germanic tribes had simply formulated soaps, as reported by Pliny the Elder. There is also some suggestion that other substances were used for cleansing, although their use would have been less extensive, and confined to particular regions. One of these substances was ox bile, which, chemically, was in some ways a forerunner of our modern synthetic detergents.

However, the primary agent in earlier days was soap. It was obtained from wood ash leached to produce potash, which, in turn, was mixed with quicklime to produce potash lye. The latter was then boiled with fat – mainly tallow – to yield soap. One major technical advance that much reduced the price of soap came early in the 19th century, when expensive potash was replaced by soda ash.

The Development of Toilet Soap

The further development of cleansing materials to produce toilet soap as we no know it came from improvements in product efficacy, emolliency, texture, and wear. One of the chief drawbacks of soap is its tendency to precipitate calcium and magnesium ions, thereby abolishing the action of the soap, as well as causing the well-known "bath-tub ring."

The search for hardness-insensitive synthetic substances therefore involved the attempt to introduce a sulphate group into an organic hydrophobic compound. In 1834, sulpholeate was obtained from sulphuric acid and olive oil; in 1875, Turkey-red oil was made from sulphuric acid and castor oil.

During World War I, IG-Farben-Industrie developed alkyl naphthalene sulphonates, which had good wetting properties but poor detergency. The situation changed when Böhme-Fettchemie, in 1928, started marketing fatty alcohol sulphates. The alkyl benzene sulphonates, first launched in 1933, remained important for many years to come as detergent ingredients. They were followed shortly afterwards, in 1935, by the alkyl phenol polyglycol ethers, which, unlike the earlier, anionic, substances, were nonionic detergents [12].

Unwanted Effects of Soap

Just as chemists were discovering new ways of formulating complex skin cleansing products, dermatologists were becoming increasingly aware that soap could be less than beneficial in certain inflammatory skin conditions. There were many studies on the subject, of which Stauffer's paper published in the Archiv für Dermatologie und Syphilis in 1930 [20] is but one example. Experimental studies in normal subjects and in eczema patients showed the former to be but little affected by soap, whereas the latter proved very sensitive, regardless of the chemical make-up of the soap employed. To quote Stauffer, "We may conclude from the results that, in general, the nature and the chemical composition of the soft soaps do not play a major role in the production of eczema; however, in subjects with an eczematous predisposition, soft soaps should be avoided since they may aggravate the eczema. This is why I tell my patients with occupational eczema not to use soft soap – a policy that has produced good results."

What, then, were these adverse effects due to? The main culprits were the alkaline pH and the calcium precipitating effect of soap exerted also in the cells of dermatitic skin and giving rise to skin irritation, exacerbation of eczema and alkali eczema. Hence the soap avoidance regimens still much quoted by textbooks of dermatology as a management principle for subjects with sensitive skin, especially those who are prone to eczema. Thus Braun-Falco, Plewig and Wolff [3] stated, in 1984, that, "Asteatotic skin tends to dry out and get irritated. Therefore, frequent or prolonged bathing or showering using alkaline soaps should be avoided."

Development of Synthetic Detergents

The crucial question in a more detailed analysis of the possible adverse biological effects – especially the skin irritation – associated with the use of soap was put by Blank [1] back in 1939, when he asked, "Is the fatty acid, the alkali or some added ingredient (perfume, dye, filler) the active etiologic agent of soap irritations?" It was known that soaps are salts of highly alkaline substances such as sodium hydroxide or potassium hydroxide and weak acids such as saturated, unsaturated or hydroxylated fatty acids. Any further development of soaps could only have come from tackling one of the possible irritants – the various fatty acids. There was nothing that could be done about the inherent – and potentially equally irritating – alkalinity of soap. Therefore, the need arose to develop novel substances. Initially, the new sulphated alcohols and sulphonated oils were used. Blank [1] described a feasible preparation of low irritancy and allergenicity, omitting dyes and perfumes (the third category of possible irritants considered by him), with a formula made up of 25% sulphonated mixed olive and teaseed oils, 25% liquid petrolatum, and 50% water. In a 2% solution, this industrially manufactured product was expected to have a pH between 6 and 7. When first used in hand eczema patients, it gave encouraging results, enabling 90% of those treated to maintain personal hygiene [1]. These results were all the more welcome as, even nowadays, it is considered vital for patients with atopic dermatitis to keep clean [15].

Surfactant development both in the United States and in Europe was held up by World War II, but caught up dramatically once the war was over. In 1947, soap accounted for 90% of the US detergent market, and synthetic detergents for 10%. Within ten years, the pattern had been reversed [19].

Initially, personal care products were not the main line of research. The story of the Maurer family in Boppard provides a good example of the way in which things evolved in Germany. In the '50's, the older brother started marketing synthetic detergents in Germany, as laundry products. In fact, it was one washing powder – REI – that gave its name to the group of companies. The products were well received by housewives. This is where the younger brother comes in. As a paediatrician, Heinz Maurer knew full well what it meant when children with a tendency towards eczema were told that they should not use soap. Impressed by the good acceptance of synthetic detergents, he suggested that the use of such substances for skin cleansing be actively explored. It rapidly became clear that such cleansing products should be made available, not only as liquids, but also in the form of solid cakes or bars, to look like good old-fashioned soap. Of course, the next question was what this novel product should be called. A synthetic cleanser bar was not the same as a bar of soap. But how should one explain that difference to the potential user?

Indications for the Use of Synthetic Detergents

Apart from a product called Praecutan Fest, the first synthetic detergent bar was "rie." This bar was tested, in the late '50's, by Keining [7] together with O. Braun-Falco and G. Weber, at the Department of Dermatology of Mainz University Hospital, to assess its action in the prevention and the treatment of various skin disorders. The lengthy list of indications established then still stands today:
1. Seborrhoeic dermatoses such as seborrhoea, acne vulgaris, rosacea, seborrhoeic dermatitis;
2. Skin disorders that rule out washing or the use of soap, such as intertrigo, dermatitis, and eczema;
3. Bacterial diseases, such as furunculosis, trichomycosis axillaris, erythrasma, as well as saprophytic or nosoparasitic mycoses such as pityriasis versicolor, candidal intertrigo, etc.

On closer scrutiny of the list, it will be seen that most of the indications are skin disorders involving increased skin wetness or oiliness, as well as skin infections. This early realization of the usefulness of acidic pH synthetic detergents in skin disorders has since been confirmed by numerous clinical reports.

Thus, Möhn and Schimpf [14] sum up their experience as follows: "The implication is that the synthetic cleanser Seba med should be used, instead of irritant products, not only in seborrhoeic disorders, different forms of hyperhidrosis, or mycotic infections (...), but especially in the subacute or chronic stages of eczematous disorders, as well as in the prevention of occupational dermatitis." Initially, the target population for the use of synthetic cleansers were adults; of late, however, these agents are being increasingly considered for use in children. In fact, studies have shown their benefit as skin care agents for infants [2].

Detergency

Prior to World War II, the detergent power of some of the candidate substances for synthetic cleansers had left much to be desired. However, the novel products that came on the market in the fifties soon proved to have superior detergency compared with conventional soaps. Studies in thousands of subjects exposed to heavy occupational soiling showed the action to be so powerful as to make industrial cleansers largely superfluous – a boon to many workers, since these cleansers had been implicated in many of the adverse skin reactions observed [18]. The superior detergency reported early on has recently been re-confirmed in studies using a skin washing simulator to cleanse artificially soiled forearm skin. Major differences were found between the synthetic cleanser seba med and the conventional-formula Lux soap, as well as between seba med and Neutrogena, a soap claimed by its manufacturers to be a neutral cleanser [24].

This powerful detergency of commercial synthetic cleansers is, of course, a mixed blessing for the dermatologist: What Modde et al. [13] said as early as 1965 still holds: "Hence dermatologists feel – at least in principle – that good detergency goes hand in hand with a high side-effect rate." This is why synthetic cleanser research nowadays is more concerned with detecting and minimizing side effects than with further enhancing the detersive action of the products.

Side Effects of Synthetic Detergents

In the '40's, methods were evolved to study the side effects of soaps. The principles then established can still be used today, to detect the side effects of synthetic cleansers. Thus, the pioneering paper by Kooyman and Snyder [9] mentions the patch test and the arm immersion test. The introduction of the unphysiological Duhring chamber test made the synthetic detergents appear worse than they are. This test which, according to Kästner and Frosch [6], correlates well with other possible methods – from the in-vitro zein test to intracutaneous testing in white mice, repeated applications to the skin of hairless mice, or the Draize rabbit eye test – makes sodium lauryl sulphate, a major ingredient of conventional synthetic cleansers, appear as a potent irritant. More recently, the Duhring chamber test has been modified to provide evidence of skin irritancy not only visually but by measurements of water vapour loss. Van der Valk et al. [23] used this method to establish a rank order of different soaps and synthetic detergent bars showing that, in terms of water vapour loss, soaps were better tolerated than cleansers. Even in its modified form, the Duhring chamber test has the disadvantage of being poorly correlated with normal use. The same criticism applies to the antecubital wash test, with which it is reported to correlate well as a rule [3]. However, the results obtained with the Duhring chamber test have, of late, prompted formulators to consider other cleanser ingredients, such as ether sulphates, amido betaines, sulphosuccinates, and isethionates [8, 17].

Neutral Synthetic Cleansers

Increasingly, another novel product category – neutral pH cleansers for "balanced" cleansing – are being marketed. Commercial cleansers nowadays tend to have a pH range from 5.0 to 7.0 [16], following Tronnier's view that, "the adjustment on the skin surface should produce a pH value of 6.4 to 6.5, rather than of 5," and that, "the drying effect of synthetic detergents is greater at pH 5 and below than if the agent is adjusted to a pH between 7 and 8." [21].

It should be noted that Marchionini and Schade's (1929) concept of the weakly acid reaction of the skin surface may, by now, be almost 60 years old, but has not been refuted by more recent experiments (cf. [4]). Most researchers still assume a mean value of 5.5; and, remarkably, Tronnier and Bussius [22] themselves found the mean pH value to be 5.8. There appears, as yet, to be insufficient experimental evidence to support the theory of the greater drying effect of synthetic cleansers of more acid pH. In order to obtain such evidence, comparative tests would have to be done using cleansers of identical formulation but differing in pH. Testing chemically disparate commercial formulations for skin roughness and oiliness [16] would not appear to be a very instructive exercise. However, a neutral pH skin cleanser may not be the ideal solution. The repeated use of acidic (pH 5.5) cleansers has been shown to result in a significantly lower skin surface pH than has repeated washing with (alkaline) soap, the corollary of the lower pH being a significantly lower skin colonization by propionibacteria [11], micro-organisms that have been held responsible for acne. It is also interesting to note that Propionibacterium acnes has a significantly lower specific growth rate at pH 5.5 than at pH values of 6.0, 6.5, or 7.0 [10].

Summary

In conclusion, it would appear that we are living in the transitional phase from the late soap age to the early synthetic detergent age. Synthetic cleansers offer more scope with regard to chemical composition, detergency, pH, and skin conditioning, and should, therefore, have a bright future.

However, there are still a number of question marks. On the one hand, the agents involved are powerful detergents. On the other, post-industrial society man is less dirty than his toiling ancestors. In the near future, therefore, the emphasis will be increasingly on such features as mildness, skin compatibility, and cosmetic acceptability.

References

1. Blank IH (1939) Action of soap on skin. Arch Dermatol 39: 811–824
2. Braun F, Lachmann D, Zweymüller E (1986) Der Einfluß eines synthetischen Detergens (Syndet) auf das pH von Säuglingen. Hautarzt 37: 329–334 (1986)
3. Braun-Falco O (1983) Letter to the editor "Test am Menschen". Ärztl Kosmetol 13: 397–406
4. Braun-Falco O, Korting HC (1986) Der normale pH-Wert der menschlichen Haut. Hautarzt 37: 125–129
5. Braun-Falco O, Plewig G, Wolff HH (1984) Dermatologie und Venerologie. 3rd ed. Springer, Berlin Heidelberg Berlin New York Tokyo, p 322
6. Kaestner W, Frosch PJ (1981) Hautirritationen verschiedener Anionen-aktiver Tenside im Duhring-Kammer-Test des Menschen im Vergleich zu In-vitro- und tierexperimentellen Methoden. Fette, Seifen, Anstrichmittel 83: 33–46
7. Keining ER (1959) Zur Frage der Reinigung gesunder und kranker Haut. Dermatol Wochenschr 140: 1245–1251
8. Koch E, Frenk E, Kligman AM (1983) Experimentelle und klinische Untersuchungen auf Hautirritationen durch Syndets. Ärztl Kosmetol 13: 11–20
9. Kooyman DJ, Snyder FH (1942) Tests for mildness of soap. Arch Dermatol 46: 846–855
10. Korting HC, Bau A, Baldauf P (1987) pH-Abhängigkeit des Wachstumsverhaltens von Staphylococcus aureus und Propionibacterium acnes. Implikationen einer In-vitro-Studie für den optimalen pH-Wert von Hautwaschmitteln. Ärztl Kosmetol 17: 41–53
11. Korting HC, Kober M, Mueller M, Braun-Falco O (1987) Influence of repeated washings with soap and synthetic detergents on pH and resident flora of the skin of forehead and forearm. Results of a cross-over trial in healthy probitioners. Acta Derm Venereol (Stockh) 67: 41–47
12. Löhr A (1963) Grundlagen des Waschvorganges. Berufsdermatosen 11: 213–230
13. Modde H, Schuster G, Tronnier H (1965) Experimentelle Untersuchungen zum Problem der Hautverträglichkeit Anion-aktiver Tenside in der Arbeitsmedizin. Tenside 2: 368–373
14. Möhn R, Schimpf A (1973) Zum "Waschverbot" bei Ekzemkrankheiten. Ther Gegenw 112: 98–102
15. Moss EM (1978) Atopic dermatitis. Pediatr Clin N Amer 25: 225–137
16. Nissen HP, Kreysel HW (1985) Flüssige Waschsyndets verschiedener pH-Wert-Einstellungen. Vergleichende Untersuchungen. Ärztl Kosmetol 15: 304–313
17. Puschmann M, Meyer-Rohn J (1983) Hautverträglichkeitsnachweis neuartiger Syndet-Präparate auf der Basis von Ethersulfaten, Amidobetainen, Sulfosuccinaten und Isäthionaten. Ärztl Kosmetol 13: 225–234
18. Schwarz HG (1964) Zur Frage des Einsatzes von Syndets anstelle von Fettseifen. Fette, Seifen, Anstrichmittel 66: 1006–1011
19. Schweinsheimer (1959) Fette, Seifen, 380; quoted in: Keining, E (1959) Zur Frage der Reinigung gesunder und kranker Haut. Dermatol Wochenschr 140: 1245–1251
20. Stauffer H (1930) Die Ekzemproben. (Methodik und Ergebnisse). Arch Dermatol Syph 162: 562–576
21. Tronnier H (1985) Seifen und Syndets in der Hautpflege und Hauttherapie. Ärztl Kosmetol 15: 19–30
22. Tronnier H, Bussius H (1961) Über die Zusammenhänge zwischen dem pH-Wert der Haut und ihrer Alkalineutralisationsfähigkeit. Z Hautkr 30: 177–195
23. Van der Valk GPM, Crejns MC, Nater JP, Bleumik E (1984) Skin irritancy of commercially available soap and detergent bars as measured by water vapour loss. Dermatosen 32: 87–92
24. Weber G (1987) A new method for measuring the skin cleansing effect of soaps and detergents. Acta Derm Venereol (Stockh) Suppl 134: 33–34

Skin Cleanser Chemistry

The Chemistry of Synthetic Detergents

Synthetic Detergents – Syndets – the Concept

K. Schumann

Terms and Definitions

Whereas soap has been around for a long time, and the "man in the street" would certainly know what soap is (even if, in all probability, he would not be able to define it), things get very much more intricate and confusing when we start looking at the detergent side of the business.

To the man in the street (or the housewife in the kitchen), a detergent is the opposite of soap. To the chemist, both soap and the modern powders or liquids are detergents (i.e. substances that have a cleaning action). While some may follow popular usage and talk of "soaps and detergents," others will refer to "synthetic detergents" to describe the modern substances.

There is, of course, also the term "surface active substances," which highlights a different property of both soaps and (synthetic) detergents, viz. their ability to alter surface tension.

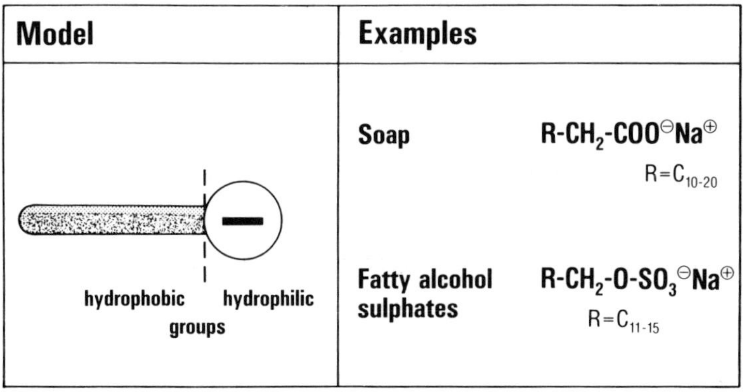

Model	Examples	
	Soap	$R\text{-}CH_2\text{-}COO^{\ominus}Na^{\oplus}$ $R = C_{10\text{-}20}$
hydrophobic — hydrophilic groups	Fatty alcohol sulphates	$R\text{-}CH_2\text{-}O\text{-}SO_3^{\ominus}Na^{\oplus}$ $R = C_{11\text{-}15}$

Fig. 1. Surfactant structure

Both "synthetic detergent" and "surface active substance" have given rise to contracted forms – "syndet" and "surfactant," respectively. While "surfactant" is very frequently used (and has, interestingly enough, been taken over as such into German for the substance that lines the pulmonary alveoli), "syndet" is less often encountered, at least in British English; in the United States, however, the (technical) cosmetics and toiletries journals are full of "syndet bars," and some articles by dermatologists use the cosmetologists' term.

German cleanser manufacturers and dermatologists have made the English term "syndet" their own, although the lay public is still largely unaware of its existence.

In German, the terminological problem was compounded for a long time by the fact that "syndet" would be used indiscriminately for the raw material (the detergent) and the finished product (the washing powder/liquid or the cleanser). In order to remedy the situation, Ernst Götte, a Düsseldorf chemist, coined a new term in 1960 to be used in Germany, and, eventually, in Europe. Referring to their action on surface and interfacial tension [1], Götte called all surface active amphiphilic substances "tensides." (There is now also a journal called *Tenside*, which has just started publication.) After careful "user testing" within Germany, the proposed term was launched at the 3rd International Congress of Surface Active Substances in Cologne, in 1964. By now, the term has become well defined, following its incorporation into the technical standards of many countries [2].

Since the "60"s, the term "syndets" has been used in Continental Europe for soap-free skin care and cleansing products. While bath and shower products also contain synthetic detergents, they are not included among the syndets. The German "Syndet" is a (toiletry) soap substitute [3], which may be solid, liquid, or a paste. Thus, the term originally used for the raw material has somehow come to mean one narrow category of products made from that raw material. It should also be noted that, unlike such terms as "soap" or "tensides," "syndets" are not covered by any definition laid down in standards.

In English, the German "Syndet" in its solid form may, as we have seen, be called a "syndet bar." There are a number of other names, such as cleanser bar, detergent bar, skin care cleansing bar, synthetic toilet bar, synthetic toilet soap; non-soap cleanser, soapless cleanser (which may, of course, be a bar or a liquid), etc. Where the context is unambiguous, the general term "synthetic detergents" may be used – as in "washing with soap and synthetic detergents."

Physical and Chemical Properties of Soap and Synthetic Detergents

Both soap and synthetic detergents chiefly contain surfactants, which means that they can reduce surface and interfacial tensions thanks to the structural principle of these substances (Fig. 1). Surfactant molecules consist of a hydrophobic and a hydrophilic part – hence the name "amphiphilic" substances. Because of this structure, surfactants (unlike, say, sugar) do not distribute themselves evenly in an aqueous medium. Apart from the molecules dissolved in the water, there will be a surfactant concentration at interfaces (e.g. the water/air interface), producing a reduction of the interfacial tension. Once the interface has been saturated, the surfactant molecules start interacting with each other to form aggregates (clusters) in the bulk phase known as micelles. These micelles are in equilibrium with the surfactant molecules at the interface and the individual molecules in the surrounding bulk phase.

These physical and chemical properties govern the use of synthetic detergents and of soap as personal cleanliness products. As a result of the adsorption and concentration of surfactant molecules at interfaces, aqueous surfactant solutions have a detersive effect, by removing poorly soluble substances from surfaces to distribute them in the body of the solution.

Whereas soap and synthetic detergents share these surfactant properties, they differ markedly in other respects. Soaps are the salts of strong alkalis and weak acids, and will produce hydroxyl ions when hydrolyzed in aqueous media. This is why soaps are alkaline by definition. Their surfactant properties are lost at neutral or acid pH. Synthetic detergents, on the other hand, have chemical structures that enable them to be surface active throughout the entire pH range (at acid, neutral, or alkaline pH values), and to be used in a "pH-controlled" manner.

Soap reacts with the hardness ions of water – chiefly Ca^{++} ions – to form poorly soluble non-detersive salts known as lime soaps ("scum"). As the salts are formed, the soap ceases to be surface active. Synthetic detergents, on the other hand, retain their surfactant properties even in very hard water. Heavy-duty or light-duty formulations can be produced, to suit different requirements. Most importantly, synthetic detergents do not form insoluble lime soaps.

Soap and Synthetic Detergents – Past and Future

Soap has been used as a cleanser for the past 4500 years. Clay tablets in cuneiform script found in Tello (in ancient Mesopotamia) describe the manufacture of a cleansing agent from oil and wood ash. Present-day soap is still made by reacting fats and oils with alkalis. Thus, the chemical principle has remained unchanged, although, of course, manufacturing technologies are now on an industrial scale [4]. To us, soap is an everyday consumer item, and few people realize that it is also a product of modern chemistry. As a toiletry item, soap has lost none of its relevance. Of the 15 million tonnes of surfactants manufactured worldwide in 1987, 8.3 million tonnes was accounted for by soap [5], most of which would have gone into body care products, with only a lesser proportion used for industrial purposes.

Nineteenth century chemists succeeded in unravelling the structure of soap; their 20th century colleagues went on to develop improved surfactants, without the inherent alkalinity and hardness sensitivity of soap. In 1928, Bertsch and Schrauth synthesized fatty alcohol sulphates to provide the first practical soap substitute [6] to go, initially, into washing powders.

The marine soaps developed in the late "30"s were the first personal cleansing bars or liquids to contain fatty alcohol sulphates, with base formulations progressing from soap-detergent combinations to pure synthetic detergent compositions. In the US and in Europe, synthetic personal care products were developed, and used side by side with conventional soap.

Table 1. Advantages of synthetic detergent cleansers

● Property	Benefit
● Hardness insensitivity	– no lime soap problems – no loss of cleansing and foaming power
● pH adjustability	– mild cleansing at neutral to acid pH levels
● Compatibility with a range of ancillary substances	– formula variability to suit different uses

Fatty alcohol sulphates are still being used as surfactants in synthetic cleansers. They have been joined by many other synthetic detergents developed over the past 60 years. Formulating chemists have succeeded in "customizing" detergents or detergent combinations that outperform conventional soap. However, almost 20 years ago, Kunstmann noted that, despite their many advantages (Table 1), synthetic cleansers could not compete with soap in the mass consumer market, although uses for such cleansers had been found in dermatology and for infant skin care. Since then, synthetic cleansers have conquered a slightly larger market share – especially in the industrialized nations – without, however, being able to rival soap, which has the significant advantage of being cheaper and of requiring manufacturing technologies that are familiar worldwide.

However, it would be inappropriate to see soap and detergents as rivals competing for the same market. They are complementary rather than mutually exclusive products. As things stand, soap will remain the dominant product for some time to come. Synthetic cleansers, however, can use a wider variety of raw materials; they can provide a wide range of properties and diversity of formulations, with more scope for innovation. As a result, the market pattern may well change sooner than expected.

References

1. Folienserie des Fonds der Chemischen Industrie 14: Tenside, Fonds der Chemischen Industrie, Frankfurt am Main, 1987
2. DIN 53900 (Juli 1972)
3. Schneider W, Thor G (1988) Hautwasch- und Reinigungsmittel. In: Umbach W (ed) Kosmetik. Thieme, Stuttgart, pp 57–79
4. Adler W, Thor G (1987) Manufacture of Bar Soap from Natural Raw Materials. In: Falbe J (ed) Surfactants in Consumer Products. Springer-Verlag, Berlin Heidelberg, pp 426–439
5. Richtler HJ, Knaut J (1988) World Prospects for Surfactants. 2nd World Surfactants Congress "Surfactants in Our World – Today and Tomorrow"
Paris 24.–27. Mai 1988
6. DE 640 997 (1928) Böhme Fettchemie
DE 659 277 (1928) Böhme Fettchemie
7. Kunzmann Th (1971) Syndetstücke und Feinseifen. Seifen–Öle–Fette–Wachse 97: 57–60

Soap – Chemical Constituents

G. Kolaczinski

Chemical Constituents of Neat Soap

Soap is produced by reacting natural fats and oils with an alkali solution.
  Soapmaking was one of the first chemical reactions performed by man [1]. The reaction product is a mixture of the alkali salts of the fatty acids used.
  The range of fats and oils for soapmaking is limited and has remained more or less unchanged for thousands of years.
  Figure 1 shows the composition of the candidate fats and oils.

It will be seen that soapmaking fats and oils fall into two categories: one containing coconut and palm kernel oils, whose chief constituent is lauric acid,

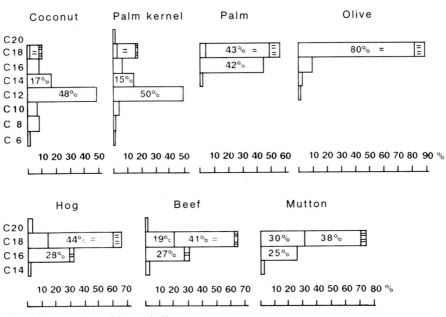

Fig. 1. Composition of fats and oils

with 12 carbon atoms; and another category of mainly C16 and C18 fatty acids, which includes palm and olive oils as well as the animal fats shown.

Initially, what went into soap was a function of local availability. Nowadays, different chain lengths are chosen to produce compositions for specific applications.

In the early Middle Ages, soapmaking flourished around the Mediterranean, with olive oil providing the chief raw material. Modern soapmakers tend to use mainly beef tallow and coconut and palm kernel oils, and, to a lesser extent, palm, peanut, and olive oils, as well as lard.

Different chain lengths of fatty acids will produce different foaming properties, and, hence, make it possible to cater for different uses. Thus, C12 and C14 soaps are quick-foaming, although the lather will be coarse and unstable; C16 and C18 soaps are slow foamers, but will produce a dense and stable lather.

Accordingly, every soapmaker will try to find his particular ideal fat base, the usual proportions nowadays being 75–85% tallow and 15–25% coconut oil.

Soap quality is influenced, not only by the fat formula adopted, but also by the quality of the raw materials, i.e. their physical and chemical properties, their colour and their odour.

The reaction of the fat mixture with the alkali solution can be produced by the conventional method of kettle soap boiling, or by the more modern industrial process of continuous saponification.

Continuous saponification relies upon preliminary fat splitting and fatty acid distillation, using the resultant fatty acid mixture for the subsequent reaction with alkali.

Either way, a neat soap containing ca. 60% fatty acids and ca. 35% water will be obtained. This substance is dried to a fatty acid content of 80%, and it is this concentrated neat soap with a water content reduced to ca. 14% that can then be used for the manufacture of toilet soap. There will still be admixtures of ca. 0.5% common salt and not more than 0.05% free alkali; after kettle boiling, there will also be between 0.5 and 1% glycerol.

Figure 2 shows a typical fatty acid chain length distribution in soap.

Additives

High quality toilet soaps are made from neat soap by the incorporation of various additives that serve to optimize the intended properties of, or impart specific features to, the soap.

Fatty Agents, Foam Stabilizers

Fatty agents are intended to counteract the defatting of the skin during washing and to give a pleasant after feel.

Foam stabilizers help to produce a rich, creamy lather. Many different substances can be employed, the usual levels varying between 1 and 10%. The

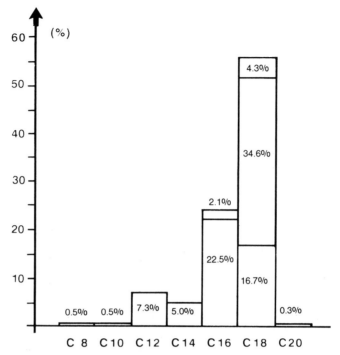
Fig. 2. Fatty acid chain length distribution

list includes free fatty acids, fatty alcohols, glycerol, lanolin, soft paraffin, cocoa butter, almond oil, wheat germ oil, as well as a range of synthetic compounds such as substituted sulphosuccinic acid esters, fatty acid isethionates, or fatty acid ethanolamides [2, 3, 4].

Of late, polymers such as Polymer JR or carbomer resins (polymer acrylates) have also been recommended for their foaming properties and emolliency [5].

Antioxidants, Sequestering Agents

Antioxidants and sequestering agents are added to soap to protect against deterioration, especially by rancidity. Soaps superfatted with – readily autoxidizable – free fatty acids are particularly prone to going rancid. Suitable agents are butylhydroxytoluene (BHT) or stearyl hydrazide. The concentrations required are between 0.02 and 0.1 %.

Sequestering agents are used to lock up the small number of heavy metal ions in the soap that can catalyze oxidative reactions. For a long time, EDTA, the sodium salt of ethylenediaminetetra-acetic acid, was used for this purpose. More recently, EHDP, ethane-1-hydroxy-1,1-diphosphonate, has become popular because of its superior action. The amounts required are between 0.1 and 0.2%.

Deodorants

Deodorant soaps came in when deodorants were evolved in the early '50's. Worries about the safety and efficacy of some of the agents initially used have led to a restriction to only 2 substances – 3, 4, 4' trichlorocarbanilide (TCC) and 2-hydroxy 2', 4,4'-trichlorodiphenyl ether (Irgasan DP-300) –, which are added singly or together, at concentrations ranging from 0.5 to 1.5%.

Colour

Most toilet soaps are dyed. Early de luxe toilet soaps came in shades of brown or olive green, presumably to mask the discoloration resulting from the addition of perfume oils. By now, many different dyes that conform to the Cosmetics Regulations are available, enabling soaps to be coloured as required by the manufacturer's product concept. Pigments are particularly suitable because of their stability. The quantities required are very small (0.01–0.05%).

Titanium dioxide is of particular importance. It is added, at levels of up to 0.2%, not only to white soaps, but also to coloured soaps to enhance their brilliance.

Under the heading of colour, mention should also be made of optical brighteners. Following increasing public concern, these agents are nowadays virtually confined to white soaps. One example is Tinopal, of which 0.01% would be required for a white soap.

Perfume Oils

The list of chemical soap constituents would be incomplete without a mention of perfume oils. The fragrances used for soapmaking must be particularly stable to discoloration and alkali. Soap manufacturers must also consider the inherent odour of the soap mass used when choosing a suitable scent [6].

Many different perfumes – complex mixtures of natural and synthetic fragrances – are used, and the list is too long to permit individual consideration. Depending on the intended use of the soap, and on its claimed position on the product scale, between 0.5 and 5% will be required. Of late, there has been a tendency to add greater rather than lesser amounts.

Special Additives

Several substances that do not come under any of the above headings are added to toilet soaps in order to impart certain performance characteristics or advertised properties; examples being milk powder, honey, chamomile extract, vitamin E, as well as abrasives for scrubbing the skin.

All additives must comply with the Cosmetics Regulations, and are therefore safe to use, in the light of present-day scientific evidence.

This survey of the chemical composition of soap shows that, apart from its main constituents – the alkali salts of fatty acids –, soap may contain a range of additives that serve to enhance its performance properties.

Soap compositions are being continually optimized. The most recent trend is towards abandoning certain agents (deodorants, optical brighteners) and marketing a largely additive-free product.

References

1. Bertrich F (1966) Kulturgeschichte des Waschens. Econ, Düsseldorf
2. Jungermann E (1985) Toilet Bar Soaps. Trends and Technologies. HAPPI 22/3: 44–48, 72, 73
3. Jungermann E (1988) An Update on Bar Soaps, Soap/Cosmetics/Chemical Specialties 6: 22–25
4. Dahlgren RM, Lukacovic MF, Michaels SE, Visscher MO (1987) Effects of Bar Soap Constituents on Product Mildness. In: Baldwin AR (ed) Second World Conference on Detergents. A.O.C.S, pp 127–134
5. Nagarajan MK (1988) New Carbomer Resins as Specicialty Additives to Toilet Soap. Seifen, Öle, Fette, Wachse 114: 589–594
6. Boeck A, Streschnak B (1988) Parfümierung kosmetischer Mittel. In: Umbach W (ed) Kosmetik. Thieme, Stuttgart, pp 332–334

Synthetic Cleansers – Chemical Constituents

W. Schneider

Traditional Soap vs. Modern Synthetic Cleansers

Synthetic cleansers belong to the more modern toiletries. They were "born" only a short while ago, quite unlike such products as soap, creams, lotions, or toothpaste that have been around for very much longer. In Germany, and in Europe as a whole, synthetic cleansers first appeared in the mid-Fifties. (Figure 1 shows an advertisement for one of the first cleanser bars marketed in Germany, featuring the novelty of the product.) At first, there were great hopes of future sales developments [1–4]. Whilst the cleansers may, perhaps, not have done as well as originally expected, they have established their position worldwide, as personal cleaning agents that share the market with soap.

However, many users still find the very product concept difficult to accept and retain. Efforts have therefore been made to develop a variety of (more or less) readily understood terms (Table 1).

Also, the chemically well-defined soaps and non-soap detergent products have by now been joined by hybrid products known as combars (combination bars), which contain different proportions of soap together with synthetic deter-

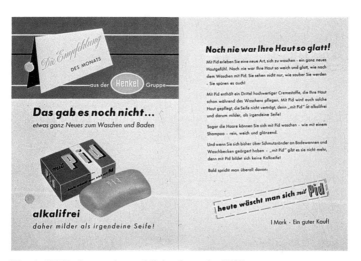

Fig. 1. "Pid" cleanser bar publicity from the "50" s

Table 1. Synonyms for synthetic cleansers

Cleanser bar	Detergent bar
Non-soap cleanser	Soap-free cleanser
Skin scare cleansing bar	"Soapless soap"
Soapless cleanser	Syndet bar
Synthetic toilet soap	Surfactant bar

gents [5]; as well as by the so-called hard water soaps, which are soaps with small amounts of lime soap dispersants added [6].

Surfactants as Main Constituents

To the consumer, a synthetic cleanser bar looks like and is used like a bar of soap, and (s)he is rarely concerned with exploring any further similarities. To the chemist, the likeness is more than "skin-deep." Both bars – the soap and the synthetic detergent one – derive their cleaning and foaming action from the surfactants contained in their formulations. These surfactants lower the surface tension, thus improving wetting, dispersing insoluble substances, producing foam, and preventing the re-aggregation of previously dispersed soil. However, it is at the level of surfactant chemistry that traditional soap differs from modern synthetic cleansers. Surfactants are classified in terms of their structure and their resultant physicochemical behaviour in aqueous media. A surfactant may be anionic, cationic, nonionic, or amphoteric [7] (Tables 2–5).

In Germany, some 380,000 tons of synthetic surfactants were used in 1987. While some of this tonnage would have gone into the making of synthetic cleansers, the bulk was used for the manufacture of washing powders, household cleaners, bath additives, shampoos, as well as for a host of industrial uses [7]. Each category of surfactants offers a wide choice. The choice of the actual agent(s) to be used will depend upon the intended use of the product, as well as on technical and economic criteria (Table 6). Usually, surfactants are not employed "straight" but as mixtures of the different categories (anionic, nonionic, amphoteric). Tables 7–9 show the types of surfactants that are found particularly frequently in synthetic cleanser formulations.

Table 2. Anionic surfactants

A hydrophobic hydrocarbon group is linked with one or two hydrophilic groups. In aqueous solutions, there is a negatively charged anion and a positively charged cation. The surfactant properties are provided by the anion.
Examples: Carboxylates, sulphates, sulphonates
– $COO^{\ominus} Me^{\oplus}$
– $OSO_3^{\ominus} Me^{\oplus}$
– $SO_3^{\ominus} Me^{\oplus}$

Table 3. Cationic surfactants

Hydrophobic and hydrophilic groups linked in the molecule. In an aqueous medium, anions and cations dissociate. The surfactant properties are provided by the cation.
Example: Quaternary ammonium compounds

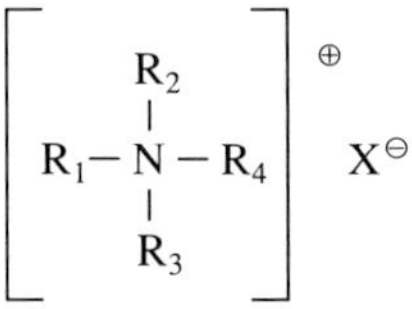

$$\left[\begin{array}{c} R_2 \\ | \\ R_1 - N - R_4 \\ | \\ R_3 \end{array} \right]^{\oplus} X^{\ominus}$$

Table 4. Nonionic surfactants

Also consist of linked hydrophobic and hydrophilic groups, but do not dissociate in aqueous media to form ions. The water solubility of these surfactants comes from interactions of the polar groups with the aqueous solvent. Examples:
Ethoxylates, alkanolamides, amine oxide

$$-O-(CH_2-CH_2-O)_n H$$

$$-CO-N \Big\langle \begin{array}{l} (CH_2-CH_2-O)_m H \\ (CH_2-CH_2-O)_n H \end{array}$$

$$\rangle N \rightarrow O$$

Table 5. Amphoteric surfactants

Hydrophobic and hydrophilic groups in the molecule. In aqueous solutions, amphoteric surfactants contain both positive and negative charges in one and the same molecule. Depending on their composition and the pH of the solution, amphoteric surfactants may have anionic or cationic properties.
Examples: Betaines, sulphobetaines

$$\rangle N^{\oplus} - CH_2 - COO^{\ominus}$$

$$\rangle N^{\oplus} - (CH_2)_n - SO_3^{\ominus}$$

Table 6. Selection criteria for surfactants to be used in synthetic cleansers

– Skin compatibility
– Biodegradability
– Lathering characteristics
– Stability to hard water
– Compatibility with other ingredients
– Consistency of raw material quality
– Processability
– Economics

Table 7. Anionic surfactants in synthetic detergents

a) Sulphates

Structure	Name
$R-CH_2-OSO_3Na$	Fatty alcohol sulphate (FAS)
$R-CH_2-O-(CH_2-CH_2-O)_n-SO_3Na$	Fatty alcohol ether sulphate (FAES)
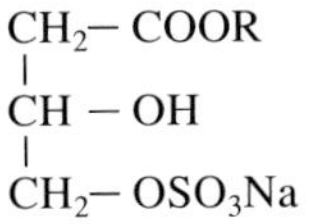 $\begin{array}{l} CH_2-COOR \\ \mid \\ CH-OH \\ \mid \\ CH_2-OSO_3Na \end{array}$	Monoglyceride sulphate

b) Sulphonates

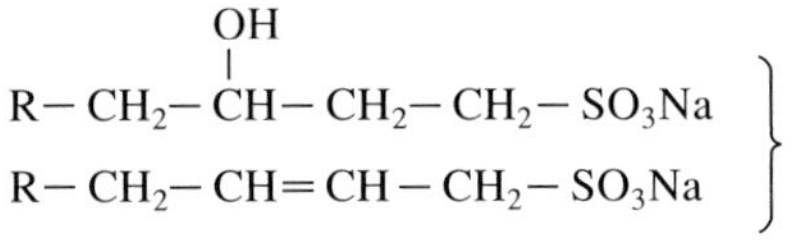

Structure	Name
$\left.\begin{array}{l} R-CH_2-\underset{\mid}{\overset{OH}{CH}}-CH_2-CH_2-SO_3Na \\ R-CH_2-CH=CH-CH_2-SO_3Na \end{array}\right\}$	Olefin sulphonate
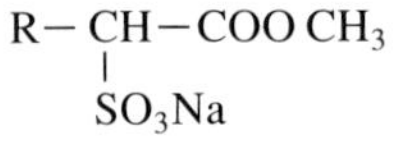 $\begin{array}{l} R-CH-COOCH_3 \\ \mid \\ SO_3Na \end{array}$	α-sulpho fatty acid ester
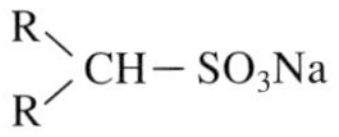 $\begin{array}{l} R \\ \diagdown \\ CH-SO_3Na \\ \diagup \\ R \end{array}$	Sec. alkane sulphonate
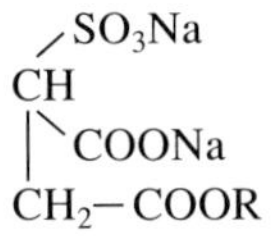 $\begin{array}{l} \diagup SO_3Na \\ CH \\ \diagdown COONa \\ CH_2-COOR \end{array}$	Sulphosuccinic acid half ester (sulphosuccinate)
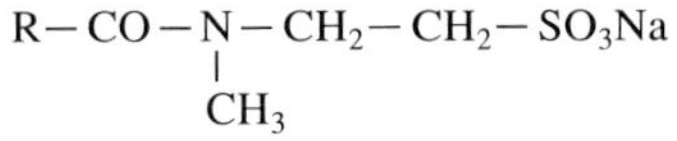 $\begin{array}{l} R-CO-N-CH_2-CH_2-SO_3Na \\ \mid \\ CH_3 \end{array}$	Methyltauride
$R-CO-O-CH_2-CH_2-SO_3Na$	Fatty acid isethionate

c) Carboxylates, phosphates

Structure	Name
$R-COONa$	Soap
$RO-(CH_2-CH_2-O)_n-CH_2-COONa$	Ether carboxylate
$\begin{array}{l} CH_3 \\ \mid \\ R-CO-N-CH_2-COONa \end{array}$	Sarcosinate
$\left.\begin{array}{l} RO-PO_3Na_2 \\ RO\diagdown \\ PO_2Na \\ RO\diagup \end{array}\right\}$	Alkyl phosphate
$\begin{array}{l} COONa \\ \mid \\ (CH_2)_2 \\ \mid \\ CH-COONa \\ \mid \\ NH-COR \end{array}$	Acyl glutamate

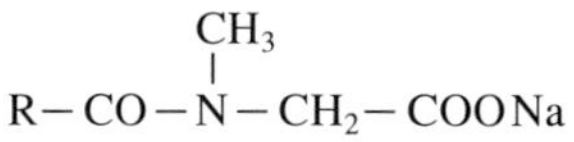

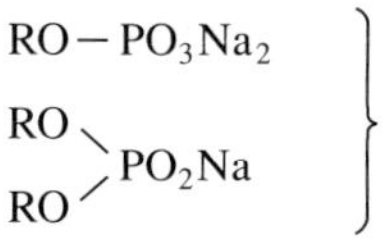

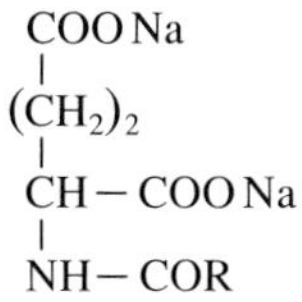

Table 8. Nonionic surfactants in synthetic detergents

$R-O-(CH_2-CH_2-O)_nH$	Polyglycol ether
$R-COO-(CH_2-CH_2-O)_nH$	Polyglycol ester
$R-CO-NH-CH_2-CH_2-OH$ $R-CO-N\big\langle{}^{CH_2-CH_2-OH}_{CH_2-CH_2-OH}$	Fatty acid alkanol amides
sugar ring with OH, OH, OH, OR, CH$_2$OH substituents	Alkyl glycosides
$R-\overset{CH_3}{\underset{CH_3}{N}}\to O$	Amide oxide

Table 9. Amphoteric surfactants in synthetic detergents

$R-\overset{CH_3}{\underset{CH_3}{N^\oplus}}-CH_2-COO^\ominus$	Alkyl betaine
$R-CONH-(CH_2)_3-\overset{CH_3}{\underset{CH_3}{N^\oplus}}-CH_2-COO^\ominus$	Alkylamidopropyl betaine
imidazolinium ring structure with $R-C$, $N-CH_2-CH_2-OH$, $N^\oplus$, $CH_2-CH_2-COO^\ominus$	Imidazolinium betaine

Other Ingredients

Making a bar of traditional soap from nothing but soap is perfectly straightforward. Trying to make a synthetic cleanser from nothing but synthetic surfactant(s) would have no user benefit other than excellent detergency – providing, of course, that such an approach were technically feasible in the first instance. This is why other ingredients have to be added to the formulation of synthetic cleansers [5, 8] (Table 10).

Table 10. Other additives

Plasticizers
Emollients/moisturizers
Fillers
pH adjusting agents
Perfume
Colour
Miscellaneous

Table 11. Plasticizers used in synthetic cleansers

Fatty alcohols
Fatty acids
Monoglycerides
Soap
Metal soaps

Table 12. Emollients/moisturizers in synthetic cleansers

Soft paraffin
Paraffin
Triglycerides
Lanolin
Lecithin

Plasticizers (Table 11) are processing aids and help to improve the structure of the finished product. They can also contribute towards the emollient properties of the cleanser. Fatty agents (Table 12) enhance the skin conditioning effect and counteract any possible harshness of the detergent. Solid fillers (Table 13) are used to improve the wear properties of the product during finishing operations and in actual use. They can also be of importance in the design of a reasonably priced cleanser. In the interest of economic viability, it should be possible to

Table 13. Fillers used in synthetic cleansers

Starch and other carbohydrates
Titanium dioxide
Talc powder
Colloidal silica
Inorganic salts

---

manufacture synthetic cleanser bars on lines normally used for soap production, which would imply similar plasticity and temperature behaviours. pH adjusting agents such as citric acid may be added to the formulation, as may fragrances, dyes, and any other ingredients specially advertised by the manufacturer. Antioxidants and sequestering agents may be beneficial, whereas preservatives are rarely used, since synthetic cleanser bars contain very little (<10%) water.

Over the last few years, various representative formulas of detergent ("syndet") bars have been published [5, 7–9].

Future Trends

In 1964, Verheggen [1] concluded that "...most of the properties of a detergent bar interact with each other. It is therefore inconceivable that one and the same bar should have maximum detergency and foaming, optimum mildness, maximum stability, best temperature stability, and greatest attractiveness, and that it should be the most reasonably priced as well." Since then, the progress made over the last 25 years is beginning to make the ideal bar a little less inconceivable.

References

1. Verheggen G (1964) Pains de toilette sans savon. Parf. Cosm. Sav. 7: 485–495
2. Manneck H (1969) Tensid-(Syndet-)Reinigungsmittel in Stückform. Seifen, Öle, Fette, Wachse 95: 467–471
3. Uzzan A (1970) Situation et avenir des détergents en barre et produits mixtes pour la toilette. Rev. Franc. Corps Gras 17: 667–672
4. Kunzmann T (1971) Syndetstücke und Feinseifen. Seifen, Öle, Fette, Wachse 97: 77–80
5. Jungermann E (1982) The Formulation and Properties of Syndet Bars. Cosm. Toil. 97: 77–80
6. Schneider W, Werner C (1980) Seifen mit verbesserten Gebrauchseigenschaften. Fette, Seifen, Anstrichmittel 82: 312–316
7. Falbe J (ed) (1987) Surfactants in Consumer Products, Springer-Verlag. Berlin, Heidelberg
8. Hollstein M, Spitz L (1982) Manufacture and Properties of Synthethic Toilet Soaps. JAOCS 59: 442–448
9. Schneider W, Thor G (1988) Hautwasch- und Reinigungsmittel. In: Umbach W (ed) Kosmetik, Thieme, Stuttgart pp 57–79

Composition of Commercial Synthetic Skin Cleansers

W. Schadenböck

Background

There are major differences in composition depending on whether the cleanser to be formulated is a solid or a liquid one.

Solid cleansers ("syndet bars") look like traditional soap. While the user may have to be told about the superior performance characteristics of the cleanser, the function and handling of the product will be obvious. Liquid cleansers are a different matter. However convincing the hygiene and application benefits of this more modern personal care product may be to the experts, users – especially in the less highly developed parts of the world – will have to go through a "learning process."

Cleanser Bars

Over the last 30 to 40 years, laundering habits have changed, with soap powders being replaced by synthetic detergent washing powders. For personal cleaning, however, toilet soap has remained dominant. This is due, partly, to the universal availability of soap, and, partly, to the cost and price differences between soap and the synthetic cleansers, which, on account of their chemical composition, will inevitably be the more expensive products.

Historical Background

The foundations for the production of solid synthetic cleansers were laid in the '30's, when Böhme AG were involved in research, and techniques had been described in US and German patents. In Germany, the first attempts at making cleanser bars go back to about 1942. In those days, Mersolat [5] (alkane and chloroalkane sulphonates) and different fillers were formulated into bars [4], using procedures (such as the co-condensation of urea and formaldehyde in the presence of Mersolat and cholesterol derivatives) that strike us, today, as mildly bizarre, and which were obviously fraught with totally unforeseeable risks.

From 1950 onwards, efforts were being made in Europe [1] as well as in the United States to develop high-quality solid cleansers to replace toilet soap. By the mid-'50's, synthetic detergent bars (or rather soap-detergent combinations) had been introduced in the United States, and were becoming increasingly popular. Products such as "Dove" and "Zest" have been going ever since.

In Germany, too, the first cleanser bars were launched in the mid-'50's. In the late '50's, the "Rie" bar was first marketed. Like its predecessors, it was based on fatty alcohol sulphates; however, it had been adjusted to a physiological (skin) pH. As a product concept, it was probably somewhat premature. Not until the launch of seba med Compact [3, 8, 2] in 1967 did cleanser bars come into their own. Since the early '80's, synthetic cleansers have been booming.

Requirements

Appearance
The bar must be smooth and flawless, its colour must be attractive, and it must be easy to handle.

Odour
The cleanser bar should have a pleasant smell that is neutral rather than pronounced. The primary function of any fragrances added should be to cover the detergent background odour.

Wear Properties, Sloughing
The mass used must be strong enough to be readily processed. Sloughing [4] – the sludging and smudging of the bar in use (a phenomenon also seen in soaps) – will be a function of the initial hardness, the water solubility, and the melting range of the bar. Sloughing should be kept to a minimum. However, since there is at least an indirect relationship between sloughing and foaming, it would not be desirable to design a completely "slough-free" bar.

Lather
Ideally, the bar should be quick-foaming and produce a dense, creamy, stable lather.

After Feel
The skin feel after use must be pleasant, smooth, and non-drying. The skin must not be excessively defatted, it must not become dull or rough. The ideal bar cleanser should leave the skin smooth, yet thoroughly cleansed.

Skin Compatibility
Use of the bar cleanser must not give rise to irritation or allergies. Obviously, as with any other product, it would be impossible to find a totally innocuous formulation. Manufacturers carry out a range of clinical studies, from patch tests to user tests over several weeks and "hypoallergenicity tests" [6] (with due consideration of the ethical aspects involved).

Typically, cleanser bars contain

- surfactants (AS, r.e. active substance)
- plasticizers/binders
- fillers
- special active ingredients
- perfumes/dyes.

Of these ingredients, the surfactants have the greatest influence on the in-use properties of the finished bar; it is also by varying this category that novel products can be designed.

Standard formula and variations

Base formula/Variation No. 1
1. Fatty alcohol sulphates (AS)	30–60%
2. Plasticizers/binders: mono-, di- and triglycerides, paraffins, microcrystalline waxes, fatty alcohols	30–50%
3. Fillers: starch, talc powder, zinc oxide, titanium dioxide	0–15%
4. Emollients/superfatting agents: lecithins, lanolin, oils, alkylol amides	1–7%
5. Special active ingredients: D-panthenol, vitamin E, amino acids, disinfectants	1–3 (10)%
6. Humectants/water: lactates, amino acids, sorbitol, glycerol	1–5%
7. Dyes	0-trace
8. Perfume	0–1%

Variation No. 2
1. Fatty alcohol sulphosuccinates (AS)	10–35%
2. Fatty alcohol sulphates (AS)	10–40%

Other ingredients as in No. 1 (2.) through (8.)

Variation No. 3
1. Fatty acid isethionates (AS)	10–40%
2. Fatty alcohol sulphates (AS)	10–40%

Other ingredients as in No. 1 (2.) through (8.)

Variation No. 4
1. Fatty acid isethionates (AS)	30–50%
2. Fatty alcohol sulphosuccinates (AS)	0–20%

Other ingredients as in No. 1 (2.) through (8.)

Variation No. 5
1. Fatty alcohol sulphates (AS), potassium salts [7]   ca. 70%
Other ingredients as in No. 1 (2.) through (8.)

In Europe, other surfactants (AS) such as lauryl sulphoacetates, acylglutamates, or taurates tend not to be used.

In Germany, and in Europe as a whole, the two main formulas are:

Formula A
ca.	50%	Fatty acid isethionates (AS)
ca.	10%	Fatty alcohol sulphosuccinates (AS)
ca.	30%	Plasticizers/binders
ca.	5%	Humectants/water
ca.	2–3%	Emollients/superfatting agents
ca.	1–2%	Special active ingredients
Remainder:		Perfumes, dyes

Formula A is the result of several years' development. The initial content of ca. 50% fatty alcohol sulphate (AS) was gradually modified to ca. 20% fatty alcohol sulphate (AS) plus ca. 30% fatty acid isethionate (AS), and eventually led to the present formulation that contains no fatty alcohol sulphates.

The actual surfactant content is roughly the same for formulations containing ca. 50% fatty alcohol sulphate and those with ca. 50% fatty acid isethionate plus 10% fatty alcohol sulphosuccinate, since the raw materials are supplied with different concentrations of surfactants (fatty alcohol sulphate >90% AS; fatty acid isethionate <80% AS).

Formula B
This base formula has remained unchanged over the years [8]; it accounts for ca. 85–99% of the finished product.

Composition
ca.	25%	Fatty alcohol sulphate (AS)
ca.	25%	Fatty alcohol sulphosuccinates (AS)
ca.	46%	Plasticizers/binders
ca.	2–5%	Water

Assuming that this base will make up 90% of the finished product, the following formulation can be derived:

ca.	23%	Fatty alcohol sulphate (AS)
ca.	23%	Fatty alcohol sulphosuccinate (AS)
ca.	42%	Plasticizers/binders
ca.	2–10%	Water
Remainder:		Emollients/superfatting agents, humectants, protein compounds, other AS (e.g. betaines), special active ingredients, perfumes and dyes.

The formulation of detergent bars requires practical experience rather than a mere textbook knowledge of the properties of each individual ingredient. The number of parameters involved is vast, and even minor departures from a previous pattern may have totally unexpected repercussions. Formulas tend to be empirical. Also, the results of laboratory tests are difficult to translate into practical terms. As a result, the development of synthetic cleanser bars is a lengthy and costly exercise.

Manufacture

In principle, synthetic cleanser bars can be produced on ordinary soap lines, using the customary mixers (kneaders), roll mills, and vacuum plodders. The smooth rod of uniform texture obtained from the plodder is cut and pressed into shaping boxes (unlike soap, which tends to be stamped); the bars thus produced may then be conditioned, or go for immediate wrapping and packaging. The mass may be mixed together from the various ingredients (powdered, melted, or dissolved raw materials); or a ready-mix base may be used, which should only require the addition of dissolved or powdered ingredients, without any melting. In either case, the subsequent finishing operations would be identical.

Liquid Synthetic Cleansers

Apart from the solid agents, (toilet soap and synthetic detergent bars), liquid synthetic cleansers are becoming increasingly popular. Liquid (conventional) soap is of very little importance.

Liquid synthetic cleansers are undoubtedly more hygienic to use, they permit easy metered dispensing, and provide wide formula variability. However, unlike bar cleansers, they require the addition of preservatives.

In Germany, liquid cleansers have been gaining a growing market share since the early '70's, and by now account for much higher sales incomes than do cleanser bars. Quite obviously, consumers are aware of the advantages offered by this product form. As with cleanser bars (seba med Compact), seba products were the pioneers of the liquid cleanser (seba med Flüssig) sector.

Composition of liquid synthetic cleansers

- surfactants (AS)
- thickeners
- emollients/mildness enhancing agents
- special active ingredients
- perfumes/dyes
- preservatives/antioxidants

Variations

Typical formulas are listed below. The concentrations quoted are "as supplied." Surfactants usually come in 30 or 40% solutions or mixtures, which means that in the finished article the AS content would be between 10 and 20% – much less than the 30–50% AS content of detergent bars.

Base formula/Variation No. 1
1. Ether sulphates, organ. neutralized (56%)(AS)	30–40%
2. Protein fatty acid condensates	0– 5%
3. Betaines (AS)	0– 5%
4. Protein hydrolysates	0– 5%
5. Thickener	1– 8%
6. Pearlizing agent	0– 5%
7. Emollients	1– 7%
8. Special active ingredients	1– 5%
9. Dyes	0-trace
10. Perfume	0–1%
11. Preservatives/antioxidants	0.05– 1% (0 in certain cases)

Variation No. 2
1. Betaines (AS)	10–40%
2. Fatty alcohol ether sulphosuccinates (AS)	10–30%
Other ingredients as in No. 1 (4.) through (11.)	

Variation No. 3
1. Betaines (AS)	10–40%
2. Protein fatty acid condensates (AS)	5–15%
Other ingredients as in No. 1 (4.) through (11.)	

Variation No. 4
1. Protein fatty acid condensates (AS)	20–50%
2. Olefin sulphonates (AS)	0–20%
Other ingredients as in No. 1 (4.) through (11.)	

Variation No. 5
1. Fatty alcohol ether sulphates (AS)	25–45%
2. Ether carboxylates (AS)	5–15%
Other ingredients as in No. 1 (4.) through (11.)	

Variation No. 6
1. Fatty alcohol ether sulphosuccinates (AS)	20–35%
2. Fatty alcohol sulphoacetates (AS)	10–15%
Other ingredients as in No. 1 (4.) through (11.)	

The following formulations are important in the liquid cleanser market:

Formula A
ca. 35% Ether sulphate, organ. neutralized (56%) (AS)
ca. 5% Protein fatty acid condensate (AS)
ca. 2% Betaines (AS)
Other ingredients as in No. 1 (5.) through (11.)

Formula B
ca. 35%Fatty alcohol ether sulphosuccinates (AS)
ca. 20%Betaines (AS)
ca. 10%Protein fatty acid condensate (AS)
Other ingredients as in No. 1 (5.) through (11.)

Formula C
ca. 30–50% Fatty alcohol ether sulphate, organ. neutralized 30% (AS)
Other ingredients as in No. 1 (4.) through (11.)

Formula D
ca. 40% Fatty alcohol ether sulphate sodium salt (AS)
ca. 10% Fatty alcohol ether sulphosuccinates (AS)
Other ingredients as in No. 1 (5.) through (11.)

Formula E
ca. 40% Fatty alcohol ether sulphate, organ. neutralized (AS)
ca. 10% Fatty alcohol ether sulphosuccinates (AS)
ca. 5% Betaines (AS)
Other ingredients as in No. 1 (5.) through (11.)

The range of (more or less) suitable candidate surfactants is vast, and the number of possible variations almost infinite. However, new products have to comply with certain requirements, such as maximum mildness; freedom from noxious substances (be they hyped-up ones like dioxane or truly toxic ones like the nitrosamines); appearance and smell. Also, the price of the cleanser must not be prohibitive. Hence, only some of the many possible formulations will lead to marketable products.

Manufacture of Liquid Cleansers

Liquid cleansers may be mixed in open or closed systems using simple equipment (rapid stirrers, anchor stirrers). Depending on the formula used, the process may consist simply of the mixing of liquid raw materials, or of the careful melting and blending of the various agents (pearlizing agents, antioxidants, thickeners). Storage and packaging are straightforward.

References

1. Blumental A (1952) Br Patent 16672/52
2. Braun-Falco O, Heilgemeir GP (1981) Syndets zur Reinigung gesunder und erkrankter Haut. Ther Gegenw 120: 1028–1045
3. Keining E (1969) Die Hautpflege mit synthetischen Detergentien. Ärztl Prax 103: 5788–5794
4. Manneck H (1969) Tensid-(Syndet-)Reinigungsmittel in Stückform. Seifen Öle Fette Wachse 13: 467–471
5. Neumüller OA (1985) Römpps Chemie Lexikon, 8th ed. p 2544: Mersolat. Franckh'sche Verlagsbuchhandlung Stuttgart
6. Shelansky HA, Shelansky MV (1953) A new technique of human patch tests. Toilet. Goods Ass. 19: 46–49
7. Tensia (Liege, Belgium) Manufacturer's publication: Klinische Erprobung von Dermactif (Tensia (NOL) 167)
8. Weber G (1968) Prüfungsbericht über seba med. Sebapharma brochure
9. Zschimmer & Schwarz. Lahnstein (BRD). Manufacturer's publication: Syndetseifenmasse Zetesap 813 A

The Use of Synthetic Detergents in Oral Hygiene Products – Effects on the Gingiva

W. Weinert

Introduction

Caries and periodontal disease are probably the most widespread disorders that afflict mankind. Both tooth decay and gum inflammation are largely due to plaque, the accumulation of bacteria, food residues, and sticky matter between the teeth.

The bacteria in the plaque, especially those that can degrade sugars, produce organic acids (chiefly lactic acid) that demineralize the tooth enamel, thereby ushering in tooth decay.

Other bacteria – mainly anaerobes – produce endotoxins that cause inflammation of the gums. This gingivitis is the first event in the sequence leading to periodontal disease.

Use of Toothpaste

Tooth decay and periodontal disease are much easier to prevent than a great many other disorders. However, for prevention to be effective, the tough, sticky, firmly adherent plaque has to be thoroughly removed. This is mainly achieved by cleaning the teeth using a brush and toothpaste. Toothpaste contains abrasives, but can also be used as a vehicle for medicinal substances that are to be applied to the teeth and gums. One of the most important substances is fluoride, which makes the enamel resistant to attack by organic acids. Toothpaste also makes the cleaning of teeth an enjoyable exercise rather than a necessary nuisance. One particularly pleasant feature of toothpaste is its foaming action. Children, especially, prefer a foaming toothpaste to a non-foaming one. This foaming action is provided by surfactants which are added to the usual constituents of toothpaste such as abrasives, medicinal substances, fluoride, preservatives, flavourings, binders, humectants, and (in certain products) colour. Table 1 shows the range of possible surfactants for use in toothpastes. Of these, sodium lauryl sulphate is by far the most frequently used worldwide. Nonionic and cationic surfactants are of very little importance in the formulation of toothpastes.

Table 1. Surfactants for use in toothpastes

Sodium lauryl sulphate
Sodium lauroyl sarcosinate
Soap
Palm kernel fatty acid surfactants
Sodium lauryl sulphoacetate
Cocomonoglyceride sulphonate
Betaines

Toothpaste Requirements Under the Cosmetics Regulation

In Germany, toothpastes (dentifrices) are considered as cosmetics. They are therefore subject to the Cosmetics Regulation rather than the Medicines Act, and have to meet the requirements of the Regulation to ensure that the ingredients used are safe. Obviously, these safety requirements will have to be met by the surfactants that go into the toothpastes. However, surfactants also have to be suitable in other respects. Thus, there are formulating requirements such as compatibility with the other constituents of toothpaste. Also, the surfactants used must not have an inherent flavour that would affect the taste of the toothpaste. It goes without saying that – like all other ingredients – the surfactants employed must comply with the most stringent purity criteria, i.e. they must be of medicinal or food quality.

Surfactants in Oral Hygiene Products

Apart from the actual *surfactants* used as foaming agents, there are surfactant-type toothpaste ingredients such as *quaternary compounds* ("quats") that are added for their antibacterial action. Among the most important agents in this group are cetylpyridinium chloride and domiphen bromide, which are used mainly in mouth washes.

Another group is constituted by the *amine fluorides*, cationic surfactants that include such substances as olaflur, hecaflur, or dectaflur, which are used to harden the enamel. In addition to this anti-caries effect, they also contribute surfactant properties. *Nonionic surfactants* are also used in toothpastes as ancillary substances to emulsify (solubilize) flavours or special active ingredients.

The main function of the surfactants is the production of foam as a result of the lowered interfacial tension. This foam helps to distribute the toothpaste constituents evenly, and assists toothbrushing by loosening plaque in the interdental spaces where toothbrushes cannot properly reach.

Through their wetting and emulsifying action, toothpaste surfactants contribute significantly to the cleaning process. This is why the surfactants themselves have been described as anti-caries substances, although (apart from a certain level of antimicrobial activity) their action is only an indirect one, through the removal of plaque.

Thus, surfactants are vitally important constituents of toothpaste to ensure protection from decay and periodontal disease.

Are Surfactants Bad for the Oral Mucosa?

Whilst the surfactants in oral hygiene products have many beneficial properties, they have been accused by some of having also adverse effects. In particular, two side effects have been alleged – damage to the oral mucosa, and alteration of food taste. The lay public, and even experts, have been perturbed by a television programme ("Monitor") on the adverse effects of surfactants – especially sodium lauryl sulphate – in toothpaste. It was claimed that, because of their surfactant properties, detergents can destroy cells, including cells of the oral mucosa. To demonstrate the effect, detergents were shown destroying red blood cells. The message was that, far from improving the condition of the gums, surfactants in dental care products would damage epithelial cells, thus giving rise to inflammation of the gums (gingivitis).

If this claim were true, toothpastes containing sufficiently high levels of surfactants should do badly in clinical tests assessing gingival parameters. However, far from doing badly, they have produced significant improvements in countless clinical studies looking at gingival parameters such as the sulcus bleeding index, gingival index, or sulcus fluid flow rate. No adverse effects on the oral mucosa have been seen when toothpastes with up to 2% surfactants were used (Fig. 1).

Studies at Freiburg University to assess the effects of different surfactants on the keratin layer of the oral mucosa also showed surfactants to be devoid of adverse effects. However, if toothpastes with substantially more than 2% surfactants are improperly used, mucosal irritation may occur. This is why the Federal Health Agency (Bundesgesundheitsamt) has laid down an upper limit of 2% for the concentration of surfactants in toothpaste. With very few exceptions, all the toothpastes on the market are below this limit; of the ones above, one is a concentrate which, if properly used, is also within the range considered as safe by the authorities.

Thus, clinical studies have shown the worries about adverse effects on the oral mucosa, and especially on the keratin layer of the mucosa, to be unfounded: The condition of the gums is not worsened but improved.

Alteration of food taste following the use of toothpastes – a phenomenon known as the "orange-juice effect" – does occur. However, this effect is brought about, not only by the surfactants in the toothpaste, but also by other constituents such as flavourings. The mechanism is not yet fully understood. However, the effect is reversible and will disappear within a short time.

In common with all other substances, surfactants may, of course, produce *allergies.* Hypersensitivity to laundry detergents, cleaners, and toiletries have been reported. However, considering the sheer volume of these substances in

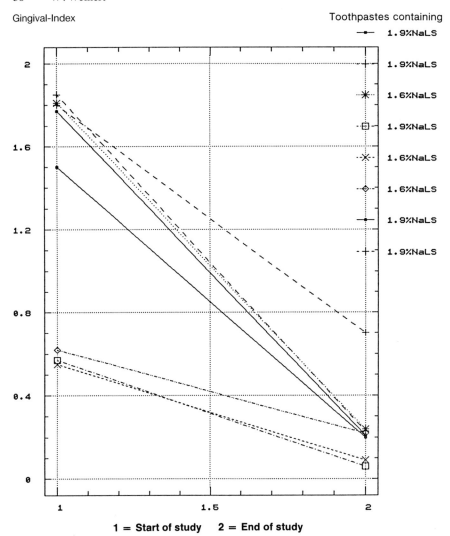

Fig. 1. Surfactant effect on gums (from [3])

everyday use, the number of adverse events is extremely small. Whilst (as with any of the products handled in everyday life) there may be the odd case of hypersensitivity to synthetic detergents, allergic reactions to toothpaste would be more likely to be due to the flavouring agents than to the surfactants contained in the product.

When toothpaste is used, small amounts will inevitably be swallowed. Studies have shown that adults may swallow about 10% of the paste put on the brush without realizing it. In children, the amounts are much greater (between 30 and

40%), while children who have not been taught to spit out after brushing, or who like the taste of the toothpaste, will swallow even more. Thus, consideration must be given to the possible systemic effects of toothpaste ingredients. Toothbrushing is a process that is repeated daily, and, consequently, it is important to know whether the long-term use of toothpaste may be harmful. Kemper (pers. communic.) states that, according to long-term studies involving much larger quantities of synthetic detergents than would be introduced by toothbrushing, the surfactants used in toothpastes are safe if used properly, even if a certain amount is swallowed.

Summary

In conclusion, surfactants are required in the formulation of toothpastes to assist the cleaning action of the product. Concentrations should be kept below 2%.

Clinical studies have provided ample evidence to show that no adverse effects on the oral mucosa need be feared, provided that the toothpaste containing the surfactants is used properly. Thus, surfactants are valuable, and, indeed, vital constituents of toothpastes.

References

1. Götze W (1977) Untersuchungen zum Einfluß von Zahnpasta auf die Gingiva. Dtsch Zahnärztl Zeitschr 32: 448–449
2. Riethe P, Schmelzle R, Schwenzer N (1980) Arzneimitteltherapie in der Zahn-, Mund- u. Kieferheilkunde. Thieme, Stuttgart
3. Seichter U (1987) Paradontopathien, Zahncremes und Natriumlaurylsulfat. Zahnärztl Mitt 77: 2253–2256
4. Vollmer G, Franz M (1985) Chemische Produkte im Alltag. Thieme, Stuttgart
5. Wallhäußer K-H (1988) Praxis der Sterilisation – Desinfektion – Konservierung. Thieme, Stuttgart
6. Die fleißigen Verbindungen. Wissenswertes über Tenside. Brochure: TEGEWA, Karlstr. 21, 6000 Frankfurt 1

Physiological and Pathophysiological Aspects of the Use of Synthetic Detergents for Skin Cleansing

Skin pH

The Physics of pH and Surface pH Measurement

H. Galster

Hydrogen Ion Activity

The importance of hydrogen ion activity in biological systems is well known. Significantly, Sørensen's pioneering treatise [11] on the definition and determination of hydrogen ion activity had the title "Enzyme Studies."

Because of the very small quantities involved, it has been customary, since then, to use the negative logarithm of the number of moles per litre, rather than the numerical value itself. This quantity is called pH, as an abbreviation of the Latin "pondus hydrogenii." As logarithms, pH values are dimensionless. The correct expression therefore would be

$$\mathrm{pH} = -\lg \frac{a_{H^+}}{a^o_{H^+}}$$

where $a^o_{H^+}$ is the standard activity of 1 mole $\cdot$ L^{-1}.

The definition of this standard activity is difficult, since activity will equal concentration only in very dilute solutions. Therefore, pH has been experimentally expressed in electrochemical terms, as the potential of a hydrogen measuring cell. However, accurate measurements can only be performed with the measuring cell used for the determination of pH standard solutions:

Ag/AgCl, KCl, standard solution, H$_2$/Pt.

The contribution of the added potassium chloride is eliminated by extrapolation to zero concentration and by the application of Debye-Hückel's theory [1].

For aqueous solutions, the pH scale ranges from 0 to 14. There is as yet no agreement on the practical definition of the scale using standard solutions. It is to be hoped that, following the latest international conference held in Stockholm in October, the thermodynamically based multi-point scale of the National Bureau of Standards (NBS) in Washington will be retained. The German DIN standard 19266 is based upon the NBS scale.

Measurement of pH

Very early on in the evolution of living beings, cells became alert to the hydrogen ion activity in their milieu. Each cell has a complex system that keeps the pH constant to within one hundredth of the target value. In a healthy subject, the pH of blood is kept to 7.414 ± 0.003, which implies a control system that by far outperforms anything that technology has so far provided.

However, since the receptors involved do not form part of our conscious sensations, we need measuring instruments in order to obtain information on pH.

In 1892, Heuß first found evidence of acidic substances in the upper layers of human skin. In the absence of more sophisticated equipment, he, like other researchers of his time, used indicators for the colorimetric determination of pH. The average value of pH = 5.5 found by Heuß in those early days still stands.

Following the advent of electrochemical methods of pH measurement, Schade and Marchionini [9] found what they called the "acid mantle" of the skin. In their work, they used a specially designed hydrogen bell electrode ("Glockenelektrode") (Fig. 1). This system gave pH values between 3.0 and 5.0, which strike us as very low in the light of more recent results. The use of the hydrogen electrode on the skin surface is fraught with particular problems that have to do with gas throughput. Unless precautions are taken against drying and carbon dioxide removal, the pH values will be affected.

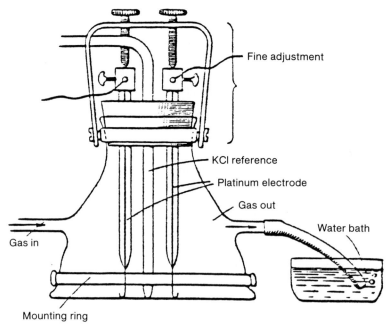

Fig. 1. Schade's bell electrode [9]. Bell diameter 5 cm

We may speculate that Marchionini might never have called the pH-stabilized layer an "acid mantle" if he had found the average value of 5.5.

Routine measurements were made possible only after Blank [2] had introduced the glass electrode into dermatology. This device, which is now used almost universally, relies upon the formation of a potential at the interface between the test solution and the glass membrane. The membrane requires activation in an aqueous solution, so that the exchange of the light alkali ions of the glass for hydrogen ions can be established in a thin layer of about 20 nm. The remaining earth alkali-silica network takes up water to form a hydrate.

This zone is often described as a "gel" – a somewhat misleading term, since the surface contains very little water, and is a gel only in a mineralogical sense, rather like opal or flint. Care must be taken to ensure that this outer layer does not dry out again. Once a glass electrode is in use, it must be kept moist.

The measuring function results from the formation of a boundary potential as equilibrium is achieved between the electrochemical potentials of the hydrogen ions in the solution and in the glass membrane. The inside of the membrane is exposed to a so-called internal buffer, whose pH provides the zero of the measuring cell. As a rule, $pH_o = 7$. The membrane potential is the difference between the pH of the test solution and that of the internal buffer. Its magnitude is governed by Nernst's equation, which, for glass electrodes, is expressed as

$$U = U_o + U'_N (pH_o - pH)$$

where U_o is the cell potential at the so-called cell zero pH_o, and U'_N is the slope of the chain.

The actual values of pH_o and U'_N are specific to the cell used, and are calibrated into the system prior to measuring by means of standard solutions. In medicine, the standards recommended by NBS may be used.

For the potential U to be measurable, the membrane glass has to have a certain electrical conductivity. This is why the earliest glass electrodes had membranes that were formed by large, thin-walled bulbs. As glasses with better conductivity came in, the fragile bulbs could be abandoned in favour of thicker-walled flat membranes, which could be applied to solid surfaces without breaking. The first reliable pH measurements using flat membrane glass electrodes (Fig. 2) were made by Schirren [13], using Polymetron cells as described by Ingold [7]. Schirren compared the results of the so-called quinhydrone electrode, which had been regarded as the most accurate before then, with the results of glass electrode measurements, on the dorsum of the hand, and found good agreement, with values of 5.17 and 5.14, respectively.

Modern electrodes are of the combination, flat membrane design shown in Figure 2. It will be seen that the system is actually made up of two electrically separate electrodes. The reference electrode is linked with the surface via the bridge solution and the porous plug or wick. Its potential is unaffected by the composition of the test medium.

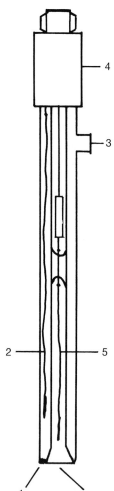

Fig. 2. Combination flat membrane electrode. *1* Porus plug, *2* Reference electrode, *3* Bridge solution filler opening, *4* Electrode cap, *5* Internal reference electrode, *6* Glass membrane

Prior to the application of the electrode, the skin must be moistened with a drop of distilled water or physiological saline. For 24 hours beforehand, the site must not be washed, and sweating must be carefully avoided.

Glass electrodes have made pH one of the more accessible parameters to be determined. Screening studies in 800 healthy subjects produced a nice, almost symmetrical Gaussian distribution (Fig. 3) [12]. The base of the curve is much wider than would be expected from the possible scatter of measurements, which suggests that the pH of human skin has a band width of at least pH = 1.5.

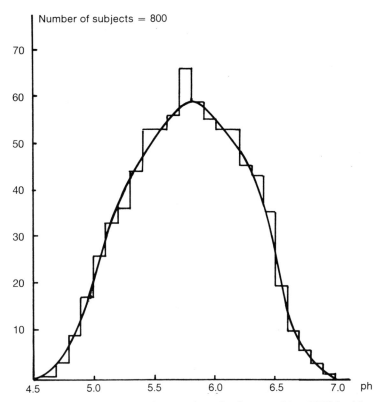

Fig. 3. Distribution of pH values on the volar forearm skin of 800 healthy volunteers; from Tronnier & Bussius [12]

Temperature Compensation

As the membrane of the glass electrode is applied to the skin, it will assume the temperature of the skin surface. Since calibration in standard solutions is usually done at room temperature, the temperature compensation of the pH meter must be manually adjusted to the surface temperature of the measuring site (e.g. 32 °C).

During prolonged measurements, or when screening several subjects in rapid succession, much of the cell will heat up, introducing errors of up to 6 mV or pH = 0.1. Since this temperature is not uniformly assumed by the entire electrode, it would be pointless to try to effect automatic temperature compensation using the built-in resistor. Care should be taken to ensure that electrodes used in dermatology are fitted with a temperature symmetrical lead, such as Bühler and Galster's "Equithal" [3].

Buffer Quality

Considering that pH is a measure of concentration, it is surprising that its measurements should be reproducible, although there are fluctuations in skin hydration and water loss, as well as different volumes of added water. This reproducibility is possible thanks to the presence, in most natural solutions, of so-called buffer systems, which control the pH of the solution concerned, ensuring constancy over a certain range in the face of dilution of, or even the addition of foreign substances to, the solution.

Apart from the carbon dioxide/sodium bicarbonate buffer system, the skin mainly relies on a system involving lactic acid and sodium lactate. A simple formula serves to illustrate the buffer function. Thus, lactic acid $CH_3CHOHCOOH$ (Hlac) dissociates according to the equilibrium

$$\frac{a_{H^+} \, a_{lac^-}}{a_{Hlac}} = K \qquad (K = 10^{-3,87})$$

Where the activity of the lactate ions a_{lac^-} may be taken to equal roughly the concentration of sodium lactate C_{lac^-}, and a_{Hlac} that of the undissociated lactic acid C_{Hlac}. In that case,

$$a_{H^+} \simeq \frac{C_{Hlac}}{C_{lac^-}} = K \qquad \text{or}$$

$$pH \simeq pK + \lg \frac{C_{lac^-}}{C_{Hlac}} \qquad (pK = 3,87)$$

The pH is close to 4, and is dependent on the lactate to free lactic acid concentration ratio. This first approximation does not contain any absolute concentrations.

Any acids or alkalis introduced from outside will change the concentrations, and, consequently, the sodium lactate to lactic acid ratio. The higher the buffer solution concentration, the less the pH will be affected. Figure 4 expresses the results of calculations to show how small amounts of alkali can be buffered, without producing any significant change in pH. Thus, a certain threshold has to be exceeded before the acid mantle of the skin will cease to function.

On average, the skin pH is slightly higher than shown in Figure 4, since, in addition to lactic acid and lactate, there is also the carbon dioxide/sodium bicarbonate buffer system operating at an optimum pH of 6.5; also, there are proteins and their degradation products, some of which, being zwitterions, can equally act as powerful buffers.

Lotmar [8] has shown how the buffer quality of the acid mantle can be determined:

With a neutral reaction, the buffer substances over a skin surface area of 24 cm^2 are dissolved within 10 min by 12 mL of a 0.004 mol · mL^{-1} sodium bicarbonate solution (pH ≈ 8), and determined by potentiometric back-titration.

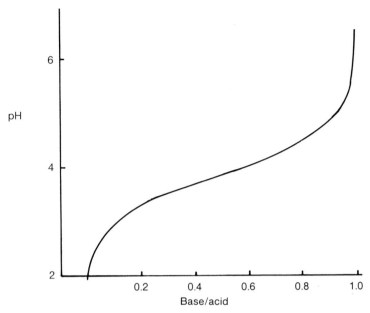

Fig. 4. Change in pH following the addition of sodium hydroxide to lactic acid

Four parameters are of importance when considering the response of the skin:

1. pH (skin pH ≈ 5.5)
2. buffer quality ($\gamma \approx 50$ nmol cm^{-2})
3. neutralizing ability ($q \approx 1$ nmol cm^{-2}s^{-1})
4. alkali resistance.

These factors come into play, one after the other, as the alkali challenge increases.

Neutralizing Ability

Any rise in pH that is not immediately compensated will stimulate the skin to produce more acid in order to restore the buffer system. Whereas pH and buffer quality are properties of the skin surface, the neutralizing ability consists in the ability of the deeper layers to send acids to the surface. Chief among these substances is the readily available carbon dioxide.

Burckhardt [4] was the first to perform quantitative measurements by placing on the skin 0.5 to 1 cm² filter paper patches soaked in 0.03 mL of a 0.0125 mol · L^{-1} sodium hydroxide solution. He then took the time to the decoloration of phenolphthalein at pH 8.3. Even after repeating the test ten times, healthy skin did not show any increase in the neutralization time.

Schneider and Tronnier [10] introduced a "modified alkali neutralization" (MAN) test, which works with a larger (4 mL) volume of 0.0005 mol $\cdot$ L^{-1} sodium hydroxide solution applied to an area of 9.25 cm^2.

With either procedure, the time of neutralization can be indicated more accurately by electrometrical means than with colorimetric indicators. Using the basic design of Burckhardt's test, the 0.03 mL drop of sodium hydroxide solution is enclosed between the skin and the glass membrane. The skin area tested is almost exactly 1 cm^2. It would even be possible to use a recorder to plot the course of pH over time.

With all these measurements, care must be taken to exclude air, since the carbon dioxide in the air would also serve to neutralize the sodium hydroxide solution. Chambers that can be strapped to the forearm (Fig. 5) have proved useful in this respect.

pH Measurements in Cosmetics and Cleansers

Creams and ointments that are oil-in-water emulsions lend themselves to direct pH measurements. All that needs ensuring is that the reference electrode is filled with liquid electrolyte and that the outflow through the membrane is at least 20 µL/d.

Many instructions recommend a dilution with a five- to ten-fold volume of distilled water.

Very greasy preparations, or pure fats, should always be emulsified prior to measuring, using a five- to ten-fold volume of distilled water. While pH measurements may be made in non-aqueous media, the value of interest is the pH that is communicated to the aqueous phase of the skin.

It will be seen that where the pH is higher than the natural 5.5 of the skin, the buffer quality of the cosmetic or cleanser becomes an important factor. It should be as low as possible so as to enable the skin to get back to its natural pH as quickly as possible.

Universally recognized pH and buffering capacity determination methods should be evolved by the German Standards Institute DIN, taking into account any international standards previously adopted in this field.

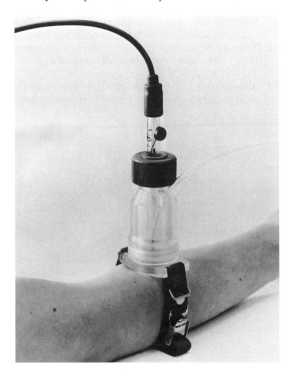

Fig. 5. Chamber for the determination of the skin's neurtralization capatity (Courtesy of Ingold Messtechnik AG, CH-8902 Urdorf)

References

1. Bates RG (1954) Determination of pH, Theory and Practice. John Wiley & Sons, New York
2. Blank KTH (1939) Measurement of the pH of the Skin Surface I. Technique. J Invest Dermatol 2: 67–74
3. Bühler H, Galster H (1985) Temperaturunabhängige Einstabmeßkette für potentiometrische Messungen. DBP 3 405 401
4. Burckhardt W (1935) Die Rolle des Alkali in der Pathogenese des Ekzems speziell des Gewerbeekzems. Arch Dermatol Syph 173: 155–167
5. DIN 19266 (1979) pH-Messung, Standardpufferlösungen. Beuth Verlag GmbH, Berlin
6. Heuß (1892) Monatsh prakt Dermatol 14: 501 (quoted in A Marchionini [1929] Untersuchungen über die Wasserstoffionenkonzentration der Haut. Arch Dermatol Syph 158: 290–333)
7. Ingold W (1951) Elektroden für die Potentiometrie und ihre Anwendungen in Laboratorium und Technik. Chimia 5: 196–203
8. Lotmar R (1964) Die potentiometrische Titration als neues Verfahren zur Bestimmung des Puffervermögens der menschlichen Haut. Arch Klin exp Dermatol 219: 610–613
9. Schade H, Marchionini A (1928) Zur physikalischen Chemie der Hautoberfläche. Arch Dermatol Syph 154: 690–716
10. Schneider W, Tronnier HZ (1958) Untersuchungen über die Einwirkungen von Schutzsalben und Waschmitteln auf die menschliche Haut unter Anwendung einer modifizierten Alkalineutralisationsprobe. Riechst.-Parfüms-Seifen 60: 6–10

11. Sørensen SPL (1909) Enzymstudien II. Über die Messung und Bedeutung der Wasserstoffionenkonzentration bei enzymatischen Prozessen. Biochem Zeitschr 21: 131–199
12. Tronnier H, Bussius H (1961) Über die Zusammenhänge zwischen dem pH-Wert der Haut und ihrer Alkalineutralisationsfähigkeit. Zeitschr Haut-Geschl Krankh 30: 177–195
13. Schirren CG (1955) Does the Glass Electrode Determine the Same pH-Values on the Skin Surface as the Quinhydrone Elektrode. J Invest Dermatol 24: 485–488

Determination of Skin Surface pH in Healthy Subjects Methods and Results of Clinical Studies

M. Kober

Background

As a subject for research, the determination of the pH of normal skin goes back to the end of the last century. Sharlit and Scheer [26] found values of around pH 5.5, which were borne out by subsequent research [18]; while other workers reported more acidic [20] or more alkaline [29] values. The literature contains a long list of methods employed in the determination of skin pH, including such techniques as colorimetry [26] or gas chain measurements using the hydrogen or quinhydrone electrodes [21]; of late [22, 15], the glass electrode originally designed by Ingold [11] has been used almost universally, since it has been found to be reliable and equal in accuracy to the quinhydrone electrode [23]. For this study (cf. [14]), it was, therefore, decided to use the latest flat glass electrode developed by Ingold to measure the pH of the skin surface.

Material and Methods

All the trials involved five male and five female healthy subjects. In order to be enrolled, candidates had to be free from skin lesions on their foreheads and the flexor side of their forearms. The average age of the subjects was 28 (range: 21–38). They were assigned to two groups, regardless of age, sex, or skin type. One group was instructed to use soap in the first instance, while the other group started washing with a synthetic detergent cleanser. The soap used was LUX toilet bar soap (Lever-Sunlicht, Hamburg); the synthetic detergent cleanser was SEBAMED-flüssig liquid cleanser (Sebapharma, Boppard). Before the trial, the pH of the two agents was tested, using the methods described below, and found to be 9.8 for LUX, and 5.59 for SEBAMED-flüssig.

For the first three days, measurements were made without the subjects using either agent. This was followed by Washing Phases I and II, each of four weeks' duration. After the baseline measurements performed during the first three days, one group started using LUX for four weeks, with a change to SEBAMED-flüssig afterwards, while the other groups started on SEBAMED-flüssig and then went on to wash with soap (cross-over design). The protocol provided for the forehead and the proximal volar forearm to be washed twice daily (mornings and evenings) for 2 minutes each time. Subjects 1–5 ("LUX group") were assigned to LUX in Phase I and to SEBAMED-flüssig in Phase II; Subjects 6–10 ("SEBAMED group") started on SEBAMED-flüssig and went on to LUX four weeks later. Forehead and forearm pH measurements were performed at strict seven-day intervals.

Apart from its short-term effect (lasting several hours), the use of skin cleansing products may also cause a considerable change in skin pH over longer periods of time [17, 27]. In order optimally to discern such long-term effects of washing with soap or synthetic detergents, the measurements were scheduled to be taken about mid-way between two washing sessions, i.e. in the afternoon. In order to obtain information also on the short-term changes in skin pH, each subject, in Phase II, underwent a single procedure of having his forehead pH taken immediately before and immediately after washing, as well as every 30 minutes during the following four hours.

The instrument used for measuring pH was a pH 521 precision pH-mV meter (WTW – Wissenschaftlich-technische Werkstätten GmbH, Weilheim), linked to a 403-S7 combination surface measuring glass electrode (Ingold, Steinbach/Ts.). The two pieces of equipment were connected using an AS7 cable made by the same company. Prior to each run, the system, after setting up and calibration, was tested repeatedly for accuracy using ready buffer solutions of pH 4.00, 4.66, 5.00, 6.00, 6.88, and 7.00 (Merck, Darmstadt). The accuracy over the range of interest was found to be at least 0.02 pH units.

During the entire trial, pH was measured as follows:
1. Before each measurement, the glass electrode was dipped, for zero calibration, into the pH 7.00 buffer; when a steady reading was obtained, the pH meter was adjusted to the value and the temperature of the buffer solution. The subsequent slope calibration was done after rinsing of the cell with bidistilled water [13, 24, 15], by dipping into the pH 4.00 buffer and setting of the slope on the pH meter. For surface measurements on the skin, a 25 °C temperature compensation setting [2] was chosen.
2. As a matter of principle, measurements at the skin sites were done three times over in order to compensate for possible fluctuations that may exist even between closely adjacent areas. For this purpose, the electrode was rinsed in bidistilled water and shaken to remove most of the water; while still slightly moist [13, 14], it was gently pressed to the middle of the forehead, above the root of the nose, and to the forearm close to the flexor crease [1, 2, 23]. Wiping the electrode with absorbent tissues had been found to be detrimental. Readings were taken when the display had steadied out, and not later than after one minute.

Since pH is, by definition, the negative logarithm to the base 10 of the hydrogen ion concentration, the pH values obtained had to be anti-logged for further calculations, to permit mean values to be derived. For the sake of clarity, the mean hydrogen ion concentrations thus obtained were then once again expressed in log form.

Data analysis was performed using standard statistical methods as described by Immich [10]. In particular, the following methods were used;
- Wilcoxon test for matched samples
- Wilcoxon test for the comparison of two independent samples.

The characteristics of the various tests were taken from the Geigy Scientific Tables [6].

Results of pH Measurements

In order to compare the baseline condition of the subject groups, forehead and forearm pH was measured on three consecutive days, at the start of the trial. The Table below shows the mean values of the subjects and of the subject groups.

Baseline pH

FOREHEAD

LUX Group

Subject No.	1	2	3	4	5	Mean	Mean overall
Day 1	4.75	4.81	4.59	5.26	4.62	4.75	
Day 2	4.49	4.97	5.53	5.29	4.52	4.79	
Day 3	4.49	4.70	5.40	5.51	5.09	4.87	4.80

SEBAMED Group

Subject No.	6	7	8	9	10	Mean	Mean overall
Day 1	4.95	4.65	4.80	4.48	5.57	4.77	
Day 2	4.81	4.51	5.05	4.53	5.56	4.76	
Day 3	5.34	4.77	5.13	4.48	5.63	4.89	4.80

FOREARM

LUX Group

Subject No.	1	2	3	4	5	Mean	Mean overall
Day 1	4.43	4.29	4.53	4.76	4.68	4.50	
Day 2	4.58	4.38	4.64	4.97	4.73	4.62	
Day 3	4.57	4.82	4.81	4.60	5.10	4.74	4.61

SEBAMED Group

Subject No.	6	7	8	9	10		
Day 1	5.23	5.04	4.22	4.70	5.02	4.68	
Day 2	5.08	4.94	4.31	4.91	5.31	4.76	
Day 3	5.44	5.39	4.47	4.81	5.05	4.88	4.77

The two groups of subjects agreed in their baseline forehead pH, while that of the forearm showed a slight discrepancy.

As will be seen from Fig. 1 (forehead) and Fig. 2 (forearm), the pH value of the LUX group rose during Phase I. This increase was followed by a considerable drop in pH when, in Phase II, SEBAMED-flüssig was used.

In the SEBAMED group, the pH remained comparatively unchanged during Phase I; this was followed by a moderate rise in pH during the LUX soap phase.

The trend seen in Figs. 3 and 4 is statistically confirmed by the Wilcoxon test. A comparison of the values of the subjects in the LUX phase (n = 10) with those of the subjects in the SEBAMED phase shows the pH to be noticeably higher when LUX soap is used (P).

The mean pH of all subjects during the LUX phase was 0.3 pH units higher than during the phase when SEBAMED was used for washing.

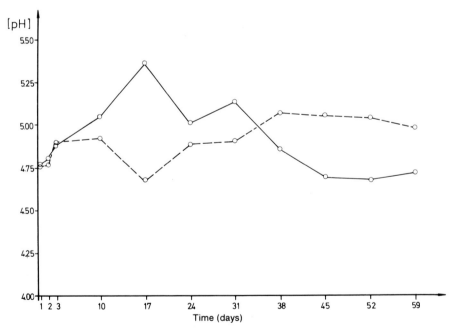

Fig. 1. Mean forehead pH vs. time in the LUX group (———) and the SEBAMED group (– – – –) (from [14])

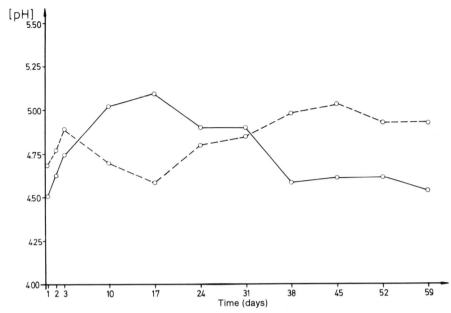

Fig. 2. Mean forearm pH vs. time in the LUX group (———) and the SEBAMED group (– – – –) (from [14])

A comparison of the corresponding weeks of all subjects – e.g. Week 1 on LUX soap vs. week 1 on SEBAMED-flüssig – for Subjects 1 through 10 shows that, with LUX soap, the pH has moved considerably into the more alkaline range (P <0.01), a trend that continues during Weeks 3 and 4 (P = 0.02).

Finally, in each group a comparison was made of the corresponding weeks of the individual subjects' washing phases (e.g. Subject No. 1 – 1st week on LUX vs. 1st week on SEBAMED-flüssig; 2nd week vs. 2nd week, etc.); the result observed above was again very clearly confirmed for both groups (P = 0.01).

The pH readings in this series were obtained immediately before and immediately after washing with the soap or the synthetic detergent. Over the following four hours, half-hourly recordings were made to study the recovery of skin pH at the washing sites.

This part of the study was carried out in Phase II for all subjects. The group who had started on LUX and were, by Phase II, using SEBAMED-flüssig had an immediate moderate rise in pH, with a return to the pre-wash level within ca. 2 hours. The other group had an immediate, very much more pronounced increase, which was also followed by a return to the pre-wash value within ca. 2 hours.

A comparison of the two groups shows that washing with either LUX soap or SEBAMED-flüssig was followed by a rise in forehead and forearm pH; however, as shown by the Wilcoxon test for two independent samples, the rise was much more pronounced in the LUX phase (P = 0.01).

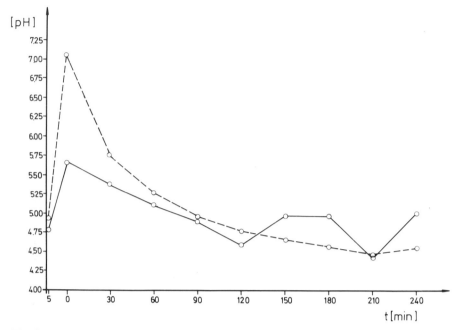

Fig. 3. Short-term courses of the mean forehead pH following the use of LUX soap (———) and of SEBAMED flüssig (– – – –) (from [14])

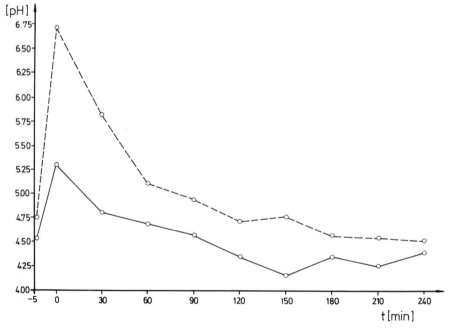

Fig. 4. Short-term course of the mean forearm pH following the use of LUX soap (———) and of SEBAMED flüssig (– – – –) (from [14])

Discussion

As pointed out by Braun-Falco and Korting [6] in their review paper, the most popular electrode for skin surface pH measurements in Germany is the flat glass electrode which was developed by Ingold in 1951, and whose equivalence with the quinhydrone electrode was shown by Schirren [23]. That these two quite different methods should yield comparable results suggests that the glass electrode (which has been in constant use to this day) gives skin surface pH values that are precise as well as accurate. In accordance with Stüttgen et al. [27], I have been able to confirm that moistening the site of electrode application is vital in order to obtain stable and reproducible measurements.

A survey of the literature readily shows that there is no such thing as a uniform pH of human skin; neither is there an accepted pH for certain sites, such as the forehead or the forearm – the sites considered in this study. I have found a mean pH of untreated forehead skin of 4.80, and of forearm skin of 4.68, with ranges from 4.49 to 5.63, and 4.22 to 5.44, respectively. At the same sites, Arbenz [2] found pHs between 5.2 and 6.8 (forehead) and 4.7 to 5.8 (forearm); Blank [5], of 4.0 to 5.6 (forehead) and 4.45 to 5.15 (forearm); and Draize [9], of 4.2 to 6.2 (forehead) and 4.2 to 5.4 (forearm).

However, as discussed above, mean pH values cannot be obtained by straightforward arithmetical operations. Also, standard deviations can be quoted only in terms of hydrogen ion concentrations and not of the logarithms of the concentrations that make up the pH scale. Most authors do not present their raw data. However, Schade and Marchionini (1928), Jolly et al. [12], and Schirren [23] do; and it will be seen, upon closer scrutiny, that their mean pH values quoted are obtained by forming the arithmetical means of the individual logarithmic data. It was therefore decided to recalculate the mean values of these authors' raw data in a mathematically unimpeachable way. This exercise produced differences by up to 0.7 units between the mean pH values quoted and the actual values obtained. Invariably – and as one would expect on purely mathematical grounds – the values quoted were too alkaline. These points are important for an understanding of my subjects' baseline pH, which may appear comparatively acidic in the light of previous ideas. Also, the earlier authors' mathematically untenable method may have prompted other researchers to assume "normal" skin pH to be somewhat more alkaline than it really is. It should also be noted that, mathematically speaking, no standard deviations can be given for pH values, although several of the earlier authors have given SDs [5, 2, 14, 4, 15, 30]. I have taken great care, in my own illustrations, to avoid presenting such information, even though this may have made the material apparently less clear.

At the start of the study, the two groups of subjects had the pH of their untreated skin measured to establish comparability. The two groups had identical mean values of 4.80 for the forehead, while for the forearm site the mean values were 4.61 and 4.77, respectively. The groups can, therefore, be taken to be fully comparable with regard to skin pH.

In general, it is considered a particular advantage for a skin cleansing agent to maintain an unaltered skin pH during use [3]. In this study, the soap (LUX soap) did not meet this requirement, while the acid pH synthetic detergent cleanser (SEBAMED-flüssig) did. With regular use of SEBAMED, the skin pH remained in its baseline range, which may be considered as a physiological one. In addition, SEBAMED abolished the relative alkalinization of the skin produced by repeated washing with LUX soap.

Not only do the two agents used differ in their long-term effects: there is also considerable difference in their short-term action. In the short term, too, washing with LUX soap produced a pronounced increase in pH that could be shown for up to two hours following exposure. The effect of washing with SEBAMED-flüssig was of the same kind, but much less in degree. Schneider [25] had found the same pH restoring effect as early as 1936. The slight, short-term alkaline shift seen with SEBAMED-flüssig may be due to the fact that even with the pH of SEBAMED-flüssig adjusted to 5.59 (vide supra), there was a slight discrepancy between the pH of the cleanser and the mean values of 4.80 and 4.68 observed in the subjects taking part in the study.

To date, there have not been any studies to investigate the effects of cleaning agents over prolonged periods of time; however, it may be concluded, in the light of the results so far obtained, that the constancy of skin pH will be affected by whether the agent used is an – inevitably – alkaline soap or a synthetic detergent cleanser that can have its pH adjusted to a value within the physiological range.

References

1. Anderson DS (1951) The acid base balance of the skin. Brit J Dermatol 63: 283–296
2. Arbenz H (1952) Untersuchungen über die pH-Werte der normalen Hautoberfläche. Dermatologica 105: 133–153
3. Athanassion AE (1964) The effects of a soap-free cleansing agent on the pH of skin. Brit J Dermatol 76: 122–125
4. Beare M, Cheeseman EA, Gailey AAH, Neill DW, Merrett JD (1960) The effect of age on the pH of the skin surface in the first week of life. Brit J Dermatol 72: 62–66
5. Blank JH (1939) Measurement of pH of the skin surface. J Invest Dermatol 2: 67–79, 231–242
6. Braun-Falco O, Korting HC (1986) Der normale pH-Wert der menschlichen Haut. Hautarzt 37: 126–129
7. Burckhardt W (1964) Methoden zur Untersuchung der Wirkung synthetischer Waschmittel auf die Haut. Dermatologica 129: 37–46
8. Geigy Scientific Tables. Geigy AG, Basel, 7th ed.
9. Draize JH (1942) The determination of the pH of the skin of man and common laboratory animals. J Invest Dermatol 5: 77–85
10. Immich H (1974) Medizinische Statistik. Schattauer Verlag, Stuttgart
11. Ingold W (1951) Elektroden für die Potentiometrie und ihre Anwendungen in Laboratorium und Technik. Chimia 5: 196–203
12. Jolly HW, Hailey CW, Netick J (1961) pH determinations of the skin. J Invest Dermatol 36: 305–308
13. Kordatzki W, Schirren CG (1952) Über eine neue Haut-pH-Meßelektrode. Klin Wochenschr 30, 840–843

14. Korting HC, Kober M, Mueller M, Braun-Falco O (1987) Influence of Repeated Washings with Soap and Synthetic Detergents on pH and Resident Flora on the Skin of Forehead and Forearm. Acta Derm Venereol (Stockh) 67: 41–47
15. Lotmar R (1958) Untersuchungen über das pH der menschlichen Haut mit besonderer Berücksichtigung seines Verhaltens nach Thermalbädern. Fundamenta Balneo-Bioclimatologica 1: 160–177
16. Peker J, Wohlrab W (1972) Zur Methodik der pH-Messung der Hautoberfläche. Dermatol Monatsschr 158: 572–575
17. Pösl H (1966) Beeinflussung des pH-Wertes der Hautoberfläche durch moderne Waschmittel, Seifen und Syndets. Thesis, Munich
18. Pösl H (1966) Beeinflussung des pH-Wertes der Hautoberfläche durch Seifen, Waschmittel und synthetische Detergentien. Hautarzt 17: 37–40
19. Rothman S (1954) Physiology and biochemistry of the skin. University of Chicago Press, Chicago, pp 221–232
20. Schade H, Marchionini A (1928) Zur physikalischen Chemie der Hautoberfläche. Arch Dermatol Syph 154: 690–718
21. Schade H, Marchionini A (1928) Der Säuremantel der Haut. Klin Wochenschr 7: 12–14
22. Schauwecker R (1955) Zur Frage der pH-Verhältnisse der nichtbefallenen Hautoberfläche bei Ekzematikern. Dermatologica 111: 197–203
23. Schirren CG (1953) Vergleichende pH-Messungen an der Hautoberfläche mit einer Chinhydron- und einer Glaselektrodenkette. Arch Dermatol Syph 197: 73–84
24. Schmid M (1952) Vergleichende Untersuchungen über die Säure-Basen-Verhältnisse auf der Haut. Dermatologica 104: 367–391
25. Schneider W (1936) Methodisches zur Bestimmung der Wasserstoffionenkonzentration. Thesis, Gießen
26. Sharlit H, Sheer M (1923) The hydrogen-ion concentration of the surface of the healthy intact skin. Arch Dermatol Syph 7: 592–598
27. Stüttgen G, Spier HW, Schwarz E (1981) Normale und Pathologische Physiologie der Haut. Springer Verlag, Heidelberg
28. Stüttgen G (1965) Die normale und pathologische Physiologie der Haut. Fischer Verlag, Stuttgart
29. Tronnier H (1985) Seifen und Syndets in der Hautpflege und -therapie. Ärztl Kosmetol 15: 19–30
30. Ude P (1978) Physikalische Hautmeßwerte und ihre topographischen Unterschiede. Ärztl Kosmetol 8: 221–227

Skin Surface pH in the Population at Large Measured Data and Correlation with Other Parameters

K. Klein, H. Evers, and H. W. Voß

Background

In 1987–88, a project involving the measurement of various skin parameters was carried out by the Health Education Research Centre of the Department of Education of Cologne University, the Gesellschaft für Umwelt, Gesundheit und Kommunikation e. V., Cologne, and the Craftsmen's Health Funds (Innungskrankenkassen).

This was the largest project of this kind ever performed in the Federal Republic of Germany. The study was done in order to establish whether the methodology used would permit the allocation of an individual to a particular skin type on the strength of a single measurement performed under normal conditions.

Material and Methods

The studies were carried out nationwide. Fig. 2 shows the sites and numbers involved. Each skin test station was equipped with an SM 410 or an SM 810 sebumeter for the determination of the skin lipid content; a CM 420 or CM 820 corneometer for the determination of skin hydration; an SMT-pH-90 pH meter; and a computer with its associated printer. A typical test station is shown in Fig. 1. The computer software supported the subject data acquisition as well as the printing of the data measured, the skin type found, and of skin care recommendations for the subject's skin type (cf. [4]). The subject data recorded were sex, age, height and weight, face care habits, occupation, and subjective well-being at the time of testing.

Measuring Method

pH measurements were made using an SMT-pH-90 pH meter (Schwarzhaupt Medizintechnik, Cologne) (cf. [5]). The equipment consisted of an electrode and the actual pH meter with a digital display (Fig. 1). Prior to each measuring run, the system has to be calibrated in two buffers (pH 4.0 and 6.9). The electrode used was of the flat glass type, and was applied to the forehead using moderate

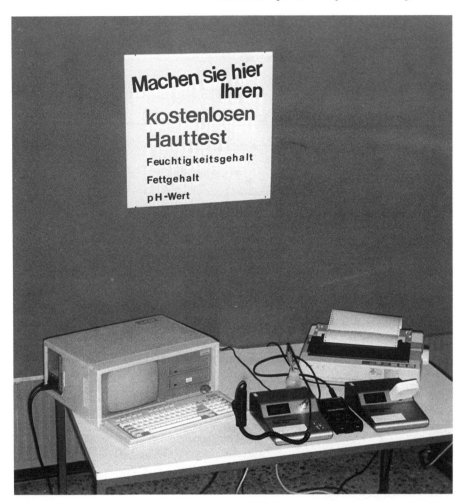

Fig. 1. Skin test station

pressure. Between measurements, the electrode was kept in distilled water. Before being used, the electrode has to be gently dried, but should be kept moist. Errors may be produced if the electrode is either too wet or too dry. In order to preclude the influence of cosmetics on the test results, subjects who had been using cosmetics heavily had their foreheads rubbed with tissues at the test station, or were excluded from the test.

The site chosen for the test was the forehead, which is sufficiently exposed to permit easy access for the investigator and minimum inconvenience for the subject being tested.

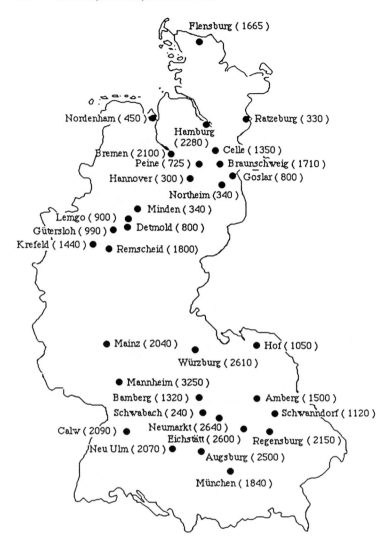

Fig. 2. Siting of skin test stations

Sample

The sample was made up of a total of 23,117 subjects (for the final analysis, there was incomplete data for some of the subjects). As will be seen from Figure 2, the study covered the whole of the Federal Republic of Germany, with test stations located not only in the cities and the major conurbations, but also in small towns and in rural areas. This approach serves to minimize possible error sources such as differences in climate, pollution levels, or regional particularities.

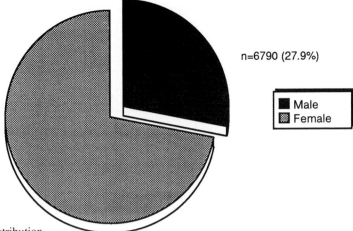

Fig. 3. Sample distribution

Figure 3 shows the breakdown of the sample by sex. Since, as a rule, the test station was open only during the day, more women than men were seen. Also, women tend to take a greater interest in skin care than do men.

Figure 4 shows the age distribution in the sample. With the exception of the Under-10 category, the pattern of the sample is about the same as that of the population at large.

The male and female populations within the sample are well matched. Table 1 shows that there is no significant difference with regard to age and the standard deviations.

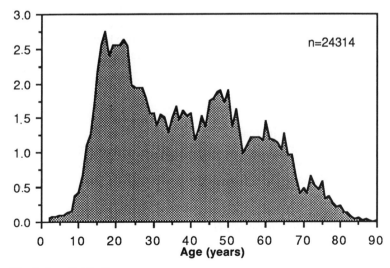

Fig. 4. Age distribution

Table 1. Comparison of the mean ages of male and female subjects

Group	Parmeter	Mean age	SD	Statistical analysis
Males		37.65	18.83	Calculated t value = 0.55 Critical t value: alpha = 0.05 beta = 0.1 t_{crit} = 1.96
Females		37.50	17.96	no significant difference

Since the number of subjects was large, good results can be obtained from all parts of the sample.

Results

Some studies performed by other workers show considerable scatter in the pH values observed, with a range in the literature from 3.5 to 6.5.

pH as a Function of Sex

Our study showed average pH values of
 4.85 for males, and
 5.00 for females.
Figure 5 shows the pH distribution within the sample as a whole.

On average, there is a difference of about 0.15 pH units between the sexes. As will be seen from Figs. 6 and 7, males have slightly lower values than do females. However, there is very little difference between the two graphs, and the two sexes may be considered as showing the same distribution.

Age and pH

Figure 8 shows an increase in pH with advancing age. Before puberty, pH values are much lower than later in life. This illustration shows a marked rise in pH during puberty (i.e. between the ages of ten and twenty), with only very little downward change in subsequent years.

Subjective Well-being and pH

pH is also a function of subjective well-being. The subjects were provided with a choice of five statements to indicate how they felt. Figure 9 shows the results

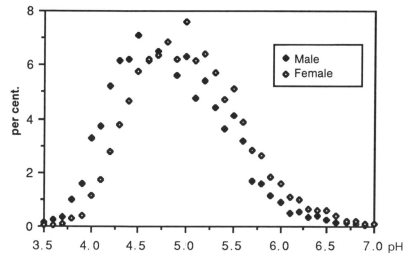
Fig. 5. pH values of male and female subjects

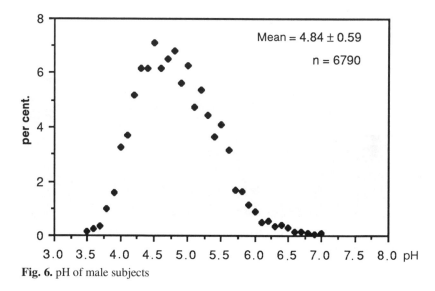
Fig. 6. pH of male subjects

of this part of the survey in relation to the pH values measured. The less well a subject felt, the higher the pH would be.

Smoking and pH

Figure 10 shows that smoking does not influence pH. The two groups were made up of smokers only and non-smokers only, respectively. Since no relevant

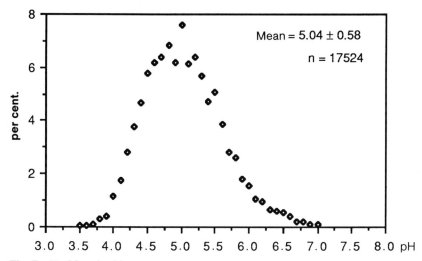
Fig. 7. pH of femal subjects

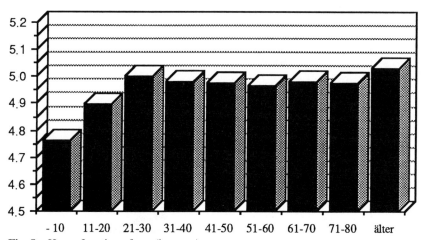
Fig. 8. pH as a function of age (in years)

difference was observed between smokers and non-smokers, no account was taken in the analysis of whether a subject had stopped smoking, or of the number of cigarettes smoked; however, the computerized questionnaire did include an item to find out whether a subject had been a smoker in the past. The significant difference found is due to the size of the sample, and would not appear to be relevant.

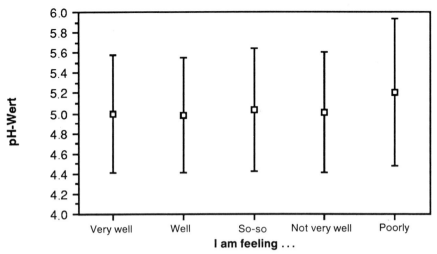

Fig. 9. Subjective well-being and pH

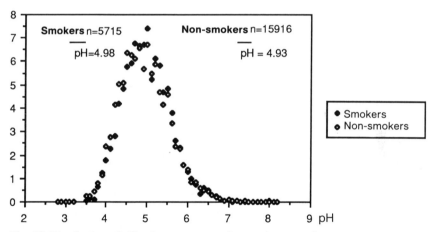

Fig. 10. Distribution of pH values among smokers and non-smokers

pH and Cosmetics

As mentioned above, cosmetics may be a source of errors. Therefore, the subjects were questioned about their use of cosmetics. Table 2 shows three different types of skin care agents and their effects on skin pH. It will be seen that, while the pH in subjects using cosmetics tends to be higher than the pH of those without any particular skin care, the influence exerted by the three types is about the same.

Table 2. Influence of different cosmetics on skin pH

Group	Mean pH	SD	Statistical analysis
No agents n = 13958	4.94	0.57	
Agents containing alcohol n = 282	5.03	0.59	p<0.05 vs. "no agents" n.s. vs. "greasy creams"
Moisturizing creams n = 6134	5.09	0.57	p<0.05 vs. "no agents" p<0.05 vs. "agents containing alcohol"
Greasy creams n = 4128	5.06	0.59	p<0.05 vs. "no agents" p<0.05 vs. "moisturizing creams"

Discussion and Summary of Results

In 1987–88, a screening study of skin surface parameters was performed nationwide (cf. [2, 3]). Since the subjects involved were healthy volunteers, their selection was entirely due to chance. Except for one age category, the sample agrees with the country's population structure.

Our values were lower than the mean of several studies quoted in the literature [1]. However, there is much scatter in the literature, with different patient populations, measuring sites, and methodologies producing very different results. Many researchers have done studies in hospitals and have therefore, in most cases, been limited to the patient material available. For technical reasons, it is usually difficult to establish a control group. Undoubtedly, earlier studies are also fraught with engineering problems since they were done with less sophisticated equipment than that available nowadays.

The reasons for the discrepancies between our results and those quoted in the literature [1] should perhaps be investigated in more detail. This paper is concerned only with a presentation of the results obtained. By now, more data has become available in this study, but is still awaiting analysis. A first, preliminary assessment would appear to confirm the results presented above.

References

1. Braun-Falco O, Korting HC (1986) Der normale pH-Wert der menschlichen Haut. Hautarzt 37: 126–129
2. Klein K, Voß HW, Voß M (1988) Untersuchungen zur Oberflächencharakteristik der menschlichen Haut Teil I. In: Umwelt und Gesundheit aktuell, Cologne
3. Klein K, Voß HW, Voß M (1988) Untersuchungen zur Oberflächencharakteristik der menschlichen Haut Teil II. In: Umwelt und Gesundheit aktuell, Cologne
4. Pohle, H, Schmitz A, Voß HW Beratungstexte aus dem Computerprogramm "Haut", Version of 07. 10. 88
5. Schwarzhaupt Skin surface pH measurement and SMT-pH-90 operating manual

Skin Flora

Principles of Bacterial Ecology

W. Dott

Terminology and Definitions

The term ecology was coined by Haeckel, in 1866, to describe the science of the household of nature. While the phase of observation, cataloguing and systematization was not yet completed, scientists went on to start the phase of causal analysis and experiments, to be followed by a third phase of systems analysis once enough data would have been provided.

Bacterial ecology is concerned with one particular aspect of ecology, that of the interrelationships among the different bacteria as well as those between the bacteria and their animate or inanimate environment.

The Ecosystem

The fundamental unit of ecology is the ecosystem. Its biotic component is the community of living organisms, also known as the biocene or biocoenosis. In bacterial ecology, this ecosystem is made up of populations of micro-organisms, with populations consisting of either a single clone of one species, or of several different species. Since bacterial cells are small (a single cell has a volume of 1 μm^3), biological function in an ecosystem will become apparent only when a certain population density of greater than 10^6 organisms has been reached.

Micro-organisms have a range of different ecosystem sizes. There are large units, e.g. aquatic areas such as rivers, lakes, sewage treatment plants; or terrestrial areas, such as the soil, or compost heaps. Equally, there are small ecosystems, e.g. the oral cavity in man, certain skin sites, the rumen of a cow, or different segments of the gut in mammals. Within each ecosystem, there will be certain environments normally occupied by certain organisms. The micro-organisms that are indigenous to a given environment are known as autochthonous. They are there because the typical conditions of the particular ecosystem provide them, more or less constantly, with the environmental conditions they require. Other micro-organisms are known as allochthonous (or zymogenous). They are only rarely found in the particular environment, or are found there only in resting forms, without playing a major role in the physiological functions normally provided by that environment.

Table 1. Abiotic factors influencing micro-organisms

Environmental factors	Growth range
Physical factors	
Temperature	−12 °C to 104 °C
Pressure	vacuum to 1400 atm
Osmolality	bidistilled water to saturated NaCl solution
Surface tension	
Radiation	UV, light, radioactivity
Gravity	
Adsorption	
Viscosity	
Chemical factors	
Water activity	a_w 1 to 0.61
pH	0 to 13
Organic nutrients	
Oxygen	0 to saturated
Redox potential	350 to 850 mV

The microbiological flora of the skin has been described as consisting of resident and of transient organisms [8]. In man, the resident flora comprises Micrococcaceae (Staphylococcus aureus, S. epidermidis, Peptococcus saccharolyticus), coryneform bacteria (Corynebacterium spp., Brevibacterium spp.) and propionibacteria (Propionibacterium acnes, P. granulosum, P. avidum). The prevalence of the different species varies between 20% and 60%. Gram-negative bacteria, among them Acinetobacter, and fungi such as Pityrosporum and Candida are also residents, although they are less often encountered [3, 5–8, 12].

The Ecological Niche

In the past, the term ecological niche was used for the actual living space of micro-organisms and the ability of the organisms to live there. Typical ecological niches of the skin flora are the perineum, the nasopharynx, the scalp, and the axilla [8]. Nowadays, the term ecological niche tends to refer to the function of a species or a population within the ecological community. This function is governed by the nutritional demands, the kinetic properties, biochemical capabilities, and structural particularities of the different organisms, as well as by their tolerance or intolerance of environmental conditions. As a rule, it will be seen that a given species or population is less widely spread than one would assume on the strength of its specific characteristics. In other words, the realized niches are usually more restricted than the preferred ones, since secondary factors will ultimately decide whether a species can utilize its potential to play its role in the community [1].

Abiotic Factors

The abiotic factors include the physical and chemical conditions of the ecosystem concerned, which influence the living conditions to which the micro-organisms are exposed. Table 1 gives a synopsis of these factors, and shows that there may be borderline areas where bacterial growth is marginally possible.

Physical Factors

Different organisms have different temperatures at which they will grow best. Biologists distinguish between psychrophiles (from Greek psychròs = cold) that like it cold; mesophiles (from Greek mésos = middle) who are fond of moderate temperatures; and thermophiles (from Greek therme = heat) who prefer high temperatures [2].
   As for higher organisms, water is vital for the growth of micro-organisms. Some of the water in a given environment may not be actually available to the micro-organisms since it will be bound by osmotic forces or by adsorption to undissolved organic matter in the water. The term water activity (a_w) has been introduced to denote water that is not bound. Water activity is defined as the vapour pressure of the medium divided by the vapour pressure of water at the same temperature.
   For the colonization of the skin by micro-organisms, the most important factors are humidity in association with temperature. An increase in either parameter can produce a ten thousand-fold increase in bacterial counts. Higher temperatures and greater humidity also bring about a shift in the microbial spectrum towards more Gram-negative organisms and coryneforms [8].

Chemical Factors

Microbes can grow within a fairly wide pH range. Some yeasts and fungi will grow even at a pH around or below 2.0. Some bacteria (Thiobacillus spp.) will produce, and can tolerate, 1N sulphuric acid. However, most micro-organisms grow best at around neutral pH. Frequent washing with soap will make the skin surface more alkaline, and favour the growth of propionibacteria [7].
   With the exception of phototrophic and lithotrophic bacteria, all organisms need to obtain their energy from the oxidation of organic substances which, under aerobic conditions, are broken down to form carbon dioxide as the end product. Under anaerobic conditions, fermentation will take place, with some of the substrate being oxidized, while another part will be excreted in the form of alcohol, acids, and aldehydes. Bacteria differ in the amount of nutrition they require from their environment. Some species (the so-called oligotrophs) can make do with very poor supplies; others (the copiotrophs) need much higher levels. In recent years, there has been much research into bacteria that can multiply under extremely nutrient-deficient conditions. There are reports of

pseudomonads being capable of multiplying in bidistilled water contaminated with trace nutrients from the air. Oligotrophs are characterized by very efficient nutrient uptake systems of high substrate affinity [9]. The supply of organic nutrients, and the physical phenomenon of adsorption, play a role in the growth of micro-organisms at interfaces. Frequently, surface films are particularly rich in ions, macromolecules, and colloidal matter, thus providing improved living conditions for micro-organisms. This is why solid surfaces and the surface film on a body of water (neuston) have particularly high bacterial counts [4]. The influence of nutrients is well illustrated by skin areas with a large number of sebaceous glands, which have a greater density of lipolytically active micro-organisms.

Biotic Factors

Table 2 gives a synopsis of the possible interactions between different micro-organisms, and between micro-organisms and higher forms of life [1, 2].

Neutralism

The term neutralism is used to describe the coexistence of two different micro-organisms, or of micro-organisms and higher life forms, in which neither is affected by the presence of the other. This can happen only if the two populations are physically separated from each other, or if they require totally different substrates.

Commensalism

Commensalism is defined as an association in which one partner derives benefit from the association while the other one derives neither harm nor benefit. One example would be the association of anaerobes and aerobes, with the aerobes rapidly reducing the oxygen content of the environment, thus making it habitable for the anaerobes. Benefit can also be provided by the excretion of growth-promoting substances (nutrients, vitamins, etc.), substrate facilitation, the neutralization of inhibitory substances, or the production of changes in the physical conditions of the habitat (pH shift, etc.). Most of the skin flora residents may be considered to be commensals.

Mutualism

There are many partnerships between micro-organisms on the one hand, and plants or animals on the other. An association in which both partners derive

Table 2. Biotic factors influencing micro-organisms

Interaction	Effect on population A	Direction of characteristic activity	Effect on population B
1. Neutralism	O	none	O
2. Commensalism	+	nutrients ←----	O
3. Mutualism (Symbiosis)	+	sometimes ←------→ direct contact	+
	+	←----→ nutrients	+
4. Antagonism			
a) Predation	+	preying ————→ ←---- nutrients	−
b) Parasitism	+	contact and ————→ penetration	−
	+	←---- nutrients	−
c) Competition	+ or −	external ←----→ nutrients	− or +
d) Amensalism	O or +	inhibitory ————→ substances	−

O = no influence, + = beneficial, − = detrimental

benefit is termed mutualism or symbiosis. There are numerous examples of syntrophism, the cross-feeding between different species of micro-organisms. Thus, bacterium A may excrete products which serve as a substrate to bacterium B but which, at higher levels, would inhibit the producing bacterium. If the two organisms live together, there will be mutual benefit, since B will be supplied with food, and will, in return, prevent A from being overwhelmed by its own products.

Antagonism

Species that live together may also harm each other, a situation that is called antagonism. There are different kinds of antagonism. The case of one species preying upon and devouring another species is known as predation. Thus, predation is confined to phagotrophic (holozoic) organisms that can ingest large particles or entire organisms. Micro-organisms such as bacteria, fungi, or algae have cell walls that prevent the ingestion of particles; they cannot, therefore, be predatory. However, it is impossible neatly to distinguish between predation and parasitism, as will be seen from the example of Bdellovibrio bacteriovorus, a bacterium which, as its name implies, eats other bacteria. This micro-organism has been variously described in the literature as a predator or a parasite [11]. Parasitism is mainly encountered in the association of micro-organisms with higher plants or animals, with the lower life form entering, and in some way harming, the higher form.

However, the association of different species of micro-organisms is more frequently characterized by competition and amensalism. In the former case, there will be rivalry, e.g. for limited food supplies, with the species that has the more efficient uptake mechanisms winning. There may also be competition among micro-organisms for binding sites. Experiments have shown that when the skin is heavily colonized by nonpathogenic strains of S. aureus, pathogenic strains of the bacterium cannot achieve adhesion. It has also been found that the systemic treatment of bacterial infections with antibiotics may lead to fungal colonization by Candida organisms.

In the latter case, that of amensalism, one species is capable of producing harmful substances that will inhibit another entity. Such substances would include antibiotics, bacteriocins, microcins, metabolic products (alcohols, organic acids, oxygen, H_2S), proteins (lytic enzymes), and phages that are temperate to population A but lytic to population B. Antibiotics are defined as microbial products which in low concentrations can inhibit or kill susceptible micro-organisms. Production of antibiotics has been observed in many micro-organisms; however, there is no agreement on the ecological importance of the phenomenon.

Microbial Ecology of the Skin

Although man's environment is teeming with micro-organisms, only few of these microbes can settle on the skin surface and multiply to form a resident population. Skin colonization starts at birth, by contact with organisms of the vaginal flora. At first, only Gram-negative and coryneform bacteria can be found. The typical pattern of predominant Micrococcaceae does not become established until later. The skin of children contains a greater variety of different species, including more pathogenic and opportunistic agents, than does the skin of adults. Propionibacteria and Pityrosporum first appear during and after puberty. There are certain sex-specific differences in microbial patterns, with men, as a rule, carrying more, and more diverse, organisms; a fact that has been attributed to their higher sweat production and more occlusive clothing. As discussed above, under physical factors, differences in temperature and humidity are responsible for different population densities at the various sites (Fig. 1). Transients are particularly numerous on exposed sites such as the face, throat, scalp, neck, and hands. The influence of the general environment on the skin

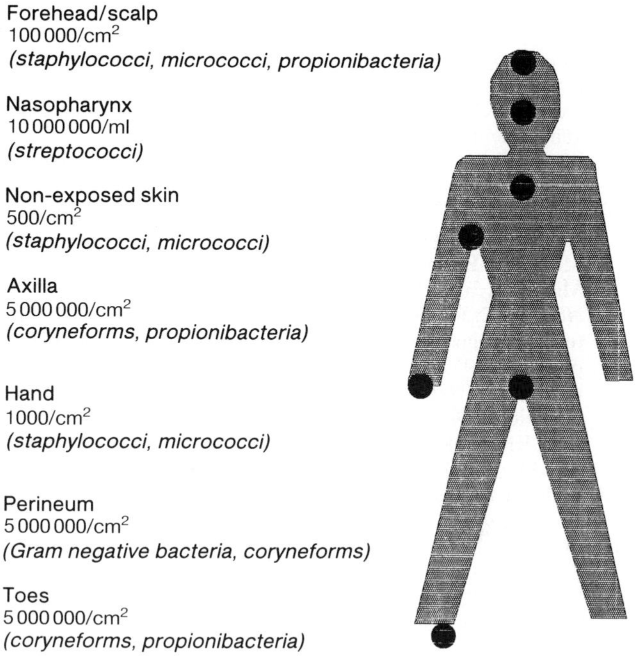

Forehead/scalp
100 000/cm^2
(staphylococci, micrococci, propionibacteria)

Nasopharynx
10 000 000/ml
(streptococci)

Non-exposed skin
500/cm^2
(staphylococci, micrococci)

Axilla
5 000 000/cm^2
(coryneforms, propionibacteria)

Hand
1000/cm^2
(staphylococci, micrococci)

Perineum
5 000 000/cm^2
(Gram negative bacteria, coryneforms)

Toes
5 000 000/cm^2
(coryneforms, propionibacteria)

Fig. 1. Ecological areas of the microbial skin flora

flora becomes particularly obvious in the hospital setting: Both hospital workers and patients have been found to carry markedly more pathogenic, opportunistic, and antibiotic resistant strains than do other subjects [3, 8, 11].

Summary

There are many possible interrelationships between micro-organisms and their environment. The pattern is characterized by the abiotic physical and chemical factors of the environment discussed above, and by the biological interactions between different species of micro-organisms as well as between micro-organisms and plants or animals. The microbial colonization of the human skin is in a state of dynamic equilibrium, with continual change in time and space. Human skin has a number of defence mechanisms (intact stratum corneum, rapid cell turnover, lipid layer, immune system) that protect against microbial overgrowth. Another defence is provided by the interference of the nonpathogenic resident flora with pathogenic transients landing on the skin. Although, normally, the association between man and microbes is one of neutralism, the pattern may turn to one of parasitism (infection) under certain circumstances (e.g. immunosuppressive therapy).

References

1. Campbell R (1977) Microbial Ecology, vol 5. Blackwell Scientific Publications Oxford London Edinburgh Melbourne
2. Doetsch RN, Cook TM (1973) Introduction to Bacteria and their Ecobiology. Medical and Technical Publishing Co. Ltd. Lancaster
3. Marshall J, Leeming JP, Holland KT (1987) The cutaneous microbiology of normal human feet. J Appl Bacteriol 62: 139–146
4. Marshall KC (1984) Microbial Adhesion and Aggregation. Springer Berlin Heidelberg New York Tokyo
5. Mok WY, Barreto da Silva MS (1984) Microflora of the human dermal surfaces. Can J Microbiol 30: 1205–1209
6. Noble WC, Pitcher DG (1978) Microbial Ecology of the Human Skin. In: Alexander M (ed) Advances in Microbial Ecology, vol 2. Plenum Press, New York London, pp 245–289
7. Peterson AF (1985) Microbiology of the Hands: Factors Affecting the Population. Rev Ind Microbiol, 26: 503–507
8. Roth RR, James WD (1988) Microbial ecology of the skin. In: In Ornston LN (ed) Ann Rev Microbiol Vol 42, Palo Alto, 441–464
9. Shilo M (1978) Strategies of Microbial Life in Extreme Environments. Verlag Chemie Weinheim New York
10. Price PB (1938) The bacteriology of normal skin. J Infect Dis 63: 301–318
11. Schlegel HG (1985) Allgemeine Mikrobiologie. Thieme Stuttgart New York
12. Skinner FA, Carr JG (1974) The Normal Microbial Flora of Man. Academic Press London New York

Composition of the Skin Flora

A. A. Hartmann

The Ecosystem of the Human Skin Flora

The flora of healthy human skin consists of *residents, temporary residents, and transients* [14, 16].

This subdivision is based upon the fact that healthy human skin is a habitat in which certain micro-organisms live together, forming an ecosystem with complex interactions, coactions, interferences, and feedbacks [14, 16, 18].

However, normal human skin is *not one single* habitat. Microbes have, as it were, a choice of *different* habitats: damp habitats in the intertriginous areas; dry habitats on the arms and legs; and sebaceous habitats on the chest, the back, in the face, and – deeper down – in the follicles of the sebaceous glands.

The habitat of the *resident* flora extends in three dimensions. These agents live on and between the corneocytes of the horny layer as well as in the sebaceous follicles, forming different size microcolonies.

Composition of Human Skin Flora

Resident Flora

Changes in the taxonomic status of members of the *resident* skin flora [1, 19] make it difficult to assess the results of skin flora ecological research from different time periods.

Qualitative Composition

In the light of today's taxonomic status of the various microbes, the following genera and species are members of the *resident* flora, i.e. they are regularly encountered on human skin:

Of the Micrococcaceae [19], the species *Staphylococcus epidermidis, S. warneri, S. haemolyticus, S. hominis, S. saccharolyticus, S. auricularis, S. saprophyticus, S. cohnii* subsp. 1; *Micrococcus agilis, M. kristinae*.

Of the genus *Propionibacterium*, the species *P. acnes, P. avidum,* and *P. granulosum*.

Of the genus *Corynebacterium*, the so-called lipophilic diphtheroids ("small colony diphtheroids") related to *Corynebacterium xerosis*; *C. pseudotuberculosis, C. kutscheri, C. pseudodiphtheriticum,* and *C. bovis.*

Of the genus *Pityrosporum* (Sloof), an imperfect fungus, the species *P. ovale* and *P. orbiculare* [11].

Quantitative Composition

It is difficult to analyze the quantities of the different genera and species that make up the *resident* flora in the different habitats, since a host of species are involved and because of the difficulty of examining single colonies grown from single samples [2]. Therefore, for staphylococci of the *resident* flora, it has been customary to use the global term "*coagulase-negative staphylococci*" to distinguish these agents from *S. aureus*, or else to use the taxonomically obsolete term "*S. epidermidis*" as proposed by Baird-Parker [1].

To illustrate the different *resident* flora patterns in different skin habitats, let us briefly look at three habitat types: dry, damp, and sebaceous.

Forearm flexor aspect (dry habitat). On the flexor aspect of the forearm, coagulase-negative staphylococci can be found, with counts of up to 10^2 to 10^3 per cm^2 of skin surface area; *lipophilic corynebacteria* are also found (10^0–10^1/cm^2). *Propionibacterium* spp. and *Pityrosporum* spp. are not found in this location [3–6, 8].

Conditions in the forearm flexor aspect habitat may be altered by wrapping the arm in cling film for 24–48 hours. As a result, the pattern of the skin flora will change: The counts of *coagulase-negative staphylococci* will rise by 3–4 powers of ten, and those of the lipophilic corynebacteria by 4–5 powers of ten. One day after the removal of the cling film, counts will still be raised, though returning towards baseline values [8]. During the occlusion with cling film, conditions in the habitat will change, with an increase in skin moisture from 20% rel. humidity to over 80% rel. humidity, while the skin pH will go from 5 to 7. One day after the removal of the cling film, these parameters will be just below the baseline values [8]. Thus, habitat conditions have a shorter recovery time than the biocene; in other words, in the human *resident* skin flora ecosystem, changes in the pattern of organisms will lag behind changes in the living conditions.

Axilla (damp habitat). There are two different patterns in this habitat: Some subjects have a microbial population dominated by *coagulase-negative staphylococci*, with *Corynebacterium* spp. of only minor importance; whereas others will show an inverse pattern [16].

Forehead (sebaceous habitat). On the forehead, *Propionibacterium* spp. account for ca. 70–90% of the residents, with counts ranging from 10^4 to 10^7 per cm^2 of skin surface area [6, 7, 9, 10, 12, 13]; *coagulase-negative staphylococci* account for ca. 10–30%, with counts from 10^2 to 10^4/cm^2; while the counts of *Pityrosporum* spp. range from 10^0 to 10^1. However, at this site, the habitat of the *resident* flora is different from the two habitats discussed above. In addition to the stratum corneum habitat, there is the one in the sebaceous follicles. Methods are available to harvest organisms separately from the two habitats [7].

The sebaceous follicles also show a differentiated distribution pattern of skin flora organisms, with *Propionibacterium* spp. along the entire depth of the follicle; *coagulase-negative staphylococci* from the middle portion of the follicle upwards; and *Pityrosporum* spp. in the uppermost part of the sebaceous gland follicle [20]. Because of this distribution in depth, it is difficult for skin disinfectants or topical antimicrobial agents to reduce the counts of the *resident* flora by more than 2 powers of ten [9, 10, 12, 13], and initial counts will be restored within 24–72 hours following the application of these agents.

Transients and Temporary Residents

Qualitative and Quantitative Composition of the Transient Skin Flora

Unlike the *resident* flora, the transients and temporary residents are seen only on the uppermost layer of corneocytes, where they will be present in low counts and for short periods of time only. This part of the skin flora includes moulds from the environment, as well as *S. aureus, Gram-negative rods* etc. Around natural body openings, there may be temporarily higher counts of organisms from the the ecosystems of the gut, the oral and the genital mucosa, and the vagina; however, these higher counts will not affect the skin.

Stabilizing Factors of the Skin Flora Ecosystem

The ecosystem of the *resident* human skin flora is largely immune to outside factors, for as long as the skin habitat is intact. Bathing once a day for three weeks, or avoidance of washing of the forearms for the same length of time, did not upset the *resident* ecosystem sufficiently to produce an overgrowth of transients [3, 4].

This comparatively great stability of the skin flora has been globally described as "*host resistance*", and has been attributed to such factors as physiological skin pH, relative skin humidity, skin lipid composition, desquamation of the stratum corneum, skin temperature, and – last but not least – to the interactions between *resident* and *transient* members of the skin flora [15, 17]. In the skin flora ecosystem, there are complex interdependences, feedbacks and multiple interactions among all these factors, which it would be extremely difficult to simulate in vitro.

References

1. Baird-Parker AC (1974) Micrococcaceae. In: Buchanan RE, Gibbons NR (eds) Bergey's manual of determinative Bacteriology 8th Ed. pp 478–490, Williams & Wilkins Company, Baltimore
2. Hartmann AA (1978) Staphylococci of the normal human skin flora. Variety in biotypes and antibiograms without direct correlation. Arch Dermatol Res 261: 295–302
3. Hartmann AA (1978) Waschverbot und Verhalten der Hautflora. Quantitative und qualitative Untersuchungen der aeroben Flora. Arch Dermatol Res 263: 105–114
4. Hartmann AA (1979) Tägliches Baden und Verhalten der Hautflora. Quantitative und qualitative Untersuchungen der aeroben Hautflora. Arch Dermatol Res 265: 153–164
5. Hartmann AA (1980) Duschbaden und sein Einfluß auf die aerobe Residentflora der menschlichen Haut. Halbseitenvergleiche unter Duschen mit und ohne Duschzusätze bei einmaliger Anwendung. Arch Dermatol Res 267: 161–174
6. Hartmann AA (1981) Zur in vitro- und in vivo-Untersuchung der Wirkung von Hautreinigungsmitteln auf die Residentflora der Haut des Menschen. Habilitationsschrift (postdoctoral thesis) Med Fac Jul-Max-Universität Würzburg
7. Hartmann AA (1982) A comparative investigation of methods for sampling skin flora. Arch Dermatol Res 274: 381–385
8. Hartmann AA (1983) Effect of occlusion on resident flora, skin-moisture and skin-pH. Arch Dermatol Res 275: 251–254
9. Hartmann AA (1985) A comparison of the effect of povidone-iodine and 60% n-propanol on the resident flora using a new test method. J Hosp Infect: 6 Suppl A: 73–80
10. Hartmann AA, Pietzsch C, Elsner P, Lange T, Hackel H, Fischer P, Bertelt T (1986) Antibacterial efficacy of Fabry's tinctura on the resident flora of the skin at the forehead. Study of bacterial population dynamics in statum corneum and infundibulum after single and repeated applications. Zbl Bakt Hyg B 182: 499–514
11. Hartmann AA (1987) Zum Stand der Taxonomie der Residentflora der Haut des Menschen. In: Hornstein O.-P. (ed) Neue Entwicklungen in der Dermatologie. Vol 4 pp 81–98, Springer, Berlin Tokyo
12. Hartmann AA, Elsner P, Lutz W, Pucher M, Hackel H (1988) Effect of the application of an anionic detergent combined with Fabry's tinctura and its components on human skin resident flora. Part I, Dermofug® combined with Fabry's tinctura and 50v/v% isopropanol. Zbl Bakt Hyg B 186: 526–535
13. Hartmann AA, Elsner P, Kremer K, Hackel H (1988) Effect of the application of an anionic detergent combined with Fabry's tinctura and its components on human skin resident flora. Part II, Dermofug® combined with salicylic acid tinctura and phenol tinctura. Zbl Bakt Hyg B 186: 536–544
14. Marples MJ (1965) The ecology of the human skin. CC Thomas, Springfield, Illinois
15. Müller E (1968) Zur Ökologie von Staphylococcus aureus auf der menschlichen Hautoberfläche der Unterarmbeugeseite und anderer Körperregionen. Arch klin exper-Dermatol 232: 350–358
16. Noble WC (1981) Microbiology of human skin. 2nd ed. In: Rook A(cons edit) Major problems in dermatology. Lloyd-Luke London
17. Röckl H (1977) Probleme der Bakterienökologie der Haut. Hautarzt 28: 155–159
18. Röckl H, Hartmann AA (1989) Mikrobenökosysteme Haut und Schleimhaut unter antimikrobieller Therapie. Z Hautkrkh (in press)
19. Schleifer KH (1986) Gram positive Cocci. In: Sneath PHA, Mair NS, Sharpe ME, Holt JG (eds) Bergey's manual of Systematic Bacteriology, Volume 2, pp 999–1103, Williams & Wilkins, Baltimore Sydney
20. Wolff HH, Plewig G (1976) Ultrastruktur der Mikroflora in Follikeln und Komedonen. Hautarzt 27: 432–440

Marchionini's Acid Mantle Concept and the Effect on the Skin Resident Flora of Washing with Skin Cleansing Agents of Different pH

H. C. Korting

Original Publications, and Comments

In 1928, A. Marchionini and his teacher H. Schade [22] published a paper in Klinische Wochenschrift entitled Der Säuremantel der Haut (nach Gasketten-messungen) (The acid mantle of the skin as determined by gas chain measurements), which contains the following statement: "We designed a 'gas chain bell electrode' adapted to the special case of the skin, a description of which is given in the more detailed paper (Arch. Dermatol. Syph. [23] H.C.K.); and were thus able to use the gas chain method for epicutaneous measurements. We would like briefly to report our results. Any preliminary cleansing, such as washing of the skin with soap, or simply rinsing with water or alcohol, must needs alter the surface reaction pattern. In order to prevent this alteration, we – unlike all previous investigators – decided to omit any 'preparatory cleansing,' and to perform our measurements on skin that had been kept clean rather than specially cleansed. To us, the response of washed skin was a problem in its own right. ... When used on the skin of living subjects, the method produced about the same high acidities (as in cadaveric skin, H.C.K.), with pH values ranging throughout from 5.0 to 3.0. Out of 40 measurements, only 2 were slightly above 5.0 ... (Fig. 1 shows a plot of the original data from Schade and Marchionini's paper, H.C.K.) Our studies have led us to the following conclusions as to the role of sweat gland secretion in the strongly acidic reaction of the skin surface: Sweat covers the skin with a very dilute solution of acids. However, as the sweat evaporates, a residue with a high acid concentration is left behind; and it is largely this fluid which impregnates the keratinizing epithelium and produces the typical high acidity of the skin surface. Thus, under normal physiological conditions, the human integument is covered with a very thin layer (mean thickness of the cornified epithelium ca. 4/100 mm) of acid, which constitutes, as it were, an 'acid mantle.' ... This phenomenon is closely related to what we consider as the most important physiological function of the acid mantle of the human skin, viz. the defence against micro-organisms in the environment. For this task, it is vital for the skin to possess the above-mentioned strikingly high acidity that we were able to detect with our gas chain measurements. ... It should be borne in mind that this defence against micro-organisms is provided, not only by the acid on the skin surface, but also by the action of sebum and by the process of continuous desquamation. It is, however, interesting to note that at

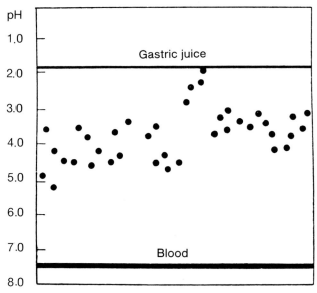

Fig. 1. Data ("Acidities of the skin surface") from the original publication by Schade and Marchionini [22]

three very different sites – the stomach, the vagina, and the skin – the body should use the same weapon – acid – to guard against microbial attack: in the stomach, the pH is 1.7–2.5 (L. Michaelis et al.); in the vagina, 4.0–4.7 (R chröder, Hinrichs and Kessler); and on the skin, about 3.0–5.0 (our measurements)."

The concept was elaborated in greater detail in a paper published by Schade and Marchionini in Archiv für Dermatologie und Syphilis [23] in 1928, with the title "Zur physikalischen Chemie der Hautoberfläche" (On the physical chemistry of the skin surface). In the same year, Marchionini also published a paper on "Untersuchungen über die Wasserstoffionenkonzentration der Haut" (Studies on the hydrogen ion concentration of the skin) [11].

A further refinement of the concept emerged ten years later, through a series of three consecutive communications published in Klinische Wochenschrift, on the general subject of the acid mantle of the skin and the defence against bacteria. The individual papers were devoted to regional differences in the hydrogen ion concentration of the skin surface [12]; regional differences in the defence against bacteria and the disinfectant powers of the skin surface [14]; and regional differences in bacterial growth on the skin surface [13]. One of the aspects studied was the time for which a micro-organism (Bacterium prodigiosum – Serratia marcescens in our modern nomenclature) placed on the skin would be able to persist in the acidic milieu of the forearm skin or the alkaline milieu of the axilla. The material Figure 2 shows is taken from the original publication (second communication).

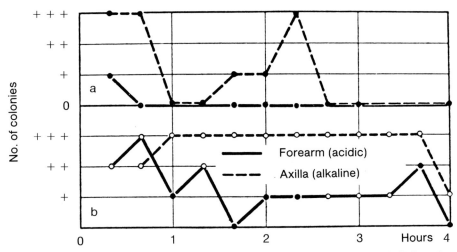

Fig. 2 a, b. Data ("Bacterial growth in acidic and in alkaline skin regions in adults") from the original publication by Marchionini et al. [14]. (**a**) Bacterium prodigiosum. (**b**) Associated flora

The idea of the acidic response of the surface of the human skin was not in itself an entirely novel one. As early as 1892, Heuss [7] had come to the conclusion, still valid today, that, "The entire skin surface of healthy subjects shows an acidic reaction, although the degree of acidity will vary depending on the site involved." Equally, in 1923, Sharlit and Scheer [25] had found a pH of 5.5 when measuring in the antecubital fossa. It was not the actual values – of between 3.0 and 5.0 – found by Marchionini that make his findings so revolutionary; indeed, the pH values reported strike us today as quite improbably acid, considering the conclusions of a recent review paper [1] that, "The analysis of all the studies quoted yields a representative (mean) pH of human skin in the range of 5.4–5.9." Where Marchionini was innovative was in his measuring technique: the use of electrodes – pioneered by him, and still the standard technique today – had been thought impossible only a few years earlier [25]. Apart from these technical innovations, Marchionini and his co-workers' outstanding contribution to science was their conclusion that the acid skin surface pH observed was related to the bacterial colonization of the skin. The term Säuremantel coined by Marchionini (variously translated into, and used in, English as "acid cloak" or "acid mantle"), however, has, at times, hampered rather than helped the cause of his idea.

The argument about the acid mantle concept and its skin bacteriological implications that is still going strong today first came to a head in the early '30's when Cornbleet [3], in his paper entitled "Self-sterilizing powers of the skin. V. Are they endowed by the surface acid?" analyzed the literature and produced his own results, with the conclusion that, "There is no proof in the literature nor do my experiments support the hypothesis that the self-sterilizing powers of the skin are due to the surface acid." In 1952, Pillsbury and Rebell [17] summed things up as follows, "The hypothesis of an 'acid mantle' as a principal factor in making the skin a less favorable area to support the growth of microorganisms has gained wide acceptance. This hypothesis is dependent upon the fact that the surface of normal unabraded skin has been shown by many observers to have a low pH. It has also been shown that intertriginous areas have a somewhat higher pH, and the conclusion was drawn that this higher pH was therefore the principal reason for the localization of infection in intertriginous areas." Pillsbury and Rebell had performed their own in-vitro experiments to study the influence of pH on the growth of different species of the skin flora [17], and found S. aureus to grow equally well at pH 5, 6 and 7; so-called normal micrococci showed somewhat but not significantly better growth at pH 6 and pH 7 than at pH 5. However, aerobic diphtheroids tended to grow significantly better at pH 7 than at lower pH levels.

Back in 1947, Foley et al. [4] made another important observation. Their in-vitro experiments showed a marked pH dependence of the fungistatic effect of different fatty acids contained in normal sweat, with different levels of activity at pH 5.0, 5.6, 6.0, and 7.0. Fatty acids such as undecylenic acid always were most effective at pH 5.0. In bacteriological studies, these results were confirmed by the observation [15] of a much greater efficacy of caprylic acid against 'Pyococcus aureus' at pH 4 than at pH 5. Along the same lines, Röckl et al. [20, 21] found that "the water soluble constituents of the horny layer" as part of a so-called preliminary overall model will kill Staphylococcus aureus and "Staphylococcus albus" at pH 5, though not at pH 7 and 8. It would also appear that the pH of the skin environment can affect not only microbial counts as such, but also the enzymatic activity of the micro-organisms. Thus, Freinkel and Shen [5] found "Corynebacterium acnes" to have, in vitro, a lipase activity at pH 7.0 that was twice as great as that at pH 5.1.

Recent Studies

The concept of the acid mantle has implications for skin cleansing, one of the main questions being whether the skin surface pH can be influenced in any major way by different cleansing methods using washing solutions of different pH. Even nowadays, many would still agree with Pillsbury and Rebell [17], who noted, in 1952, that, "These experiments (treating patients with emulsions of different pH, H.C.K.) did nothing but give further evidence of the marked and admirable capacity of the skin surface to tolerate wide variations in pH." Most studies must remain inconclusive because they were concerned solely with investigating the effects of a single application of a skin cleansing agent, be it soap [15] or a synthetic detergent [2].

One study that went beyond an investigation of the effects of a single application, to consider what happened with the repeated use of soaps or synthetic cleansers, was done by Pösl and Schirren [18]. Following a single application of a traditional soap (e.g. LUX) solution, the authors found a rise in pH by about 2 units, to pH 7.5; when an acidic synthetic detergent such as RIE was used, they found the effect to be "strikingly low" (without specifying what that meant). The question of kinetics is covered by the summary statement that, "Four hours after the end of exposure, the pH was again markedly decreased; in some cases, it had, by then, gone back to the pre-exposure value." The situation following the repeated use of LUX soap solution is described by Pösl and Schirren as follows: "The morning baseline values on the following days (Day 2 and Day 3), on which the subjects were exposed to soap solution 3 times within a 12-hour period, were a little more alkaline." However, the authors' conclusion is that, "Synthetic detergents have a less alkaline pH than do traditional toilet soap and laundry powder solutions. They will, therefore, have less effect on the pH of the skin surface. However, even repeated alkali exposure, using either synthetic detergents or conventional soap or laundry agent solutions three times a day, for half an hour at a time, over a period of 3–5 days, will not produce a lasting alteration of the alkaline skin surface pH or an exhaustion of the skin's buffering capacity."

There are few investigations into the effect of repeated washing on the bacterial flora of the skin; most of the interest appears to have been not in simple (hand) washing, but in bathing [8] or showering [6]. Such studies as have been performed have not looked at pH. It therefore appeared vital to see what happened to skin surface pH and the resident bacterial flora in a study involving the repeated use, over an extended period and under well-defined conditions, of soap and a synthetic detergent cleanser.

Our Skin Cleanser Studies

The study involved a total of 10 subjects with healthy skin. For the first three days, while the subjects were continuing their previous skin cleansing practices, skin pH and the densities of coagulase-negative staphylococci and propionibacteria were repeatedly determined on the forehead (centre) and the forearm (distal to the antecubital fossa) [10]. Five of the subjects then spent four weeks washing with an (alkaline) soap (LUX soap, Lever, Hamburg, FRG), mornings and evenings, each washing session lasting two minutes. The five others were asked to carry out the same protocol, using an acid pH synthetic detergent solution (seba med flüssig, Sebapharma, Boppard, FRG). After four weeks, the subjects were crossed over, for another period of four weeks. At the end of each week, skin pH and the bacterial flora were determined in the interval between washings, at least four hours after the last washing session. For pH measurements, the method described by Schirren [24] with an Ingold flat glass electrode was used. Microbial counts were done in material obtained by the detergent scrub method described by Williamson and Kligman [26]. Serial dilutions were inoculated onto Columbia agar (BBL, Heidelberg, FRG) with 5% defibrinated sheep blood and trypticase soy agar (BBL), with incubation for two and seven days, respectively, at 37°C, under aerobic or anaerobic (GasPak jars, BBL) conditions. Coagulase-negative staphylococci were identified by means of Gram staining,

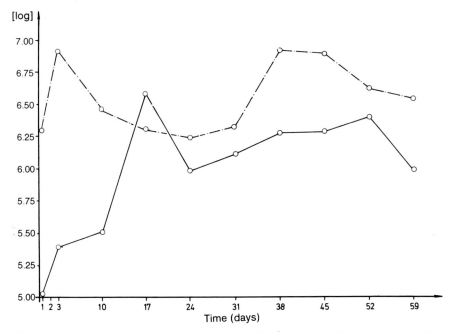

Fig. 3. Counts of coagulase-negative staphylococci/cm^2 forehead skin vs. time (*solid line* = soap first) (from [10])

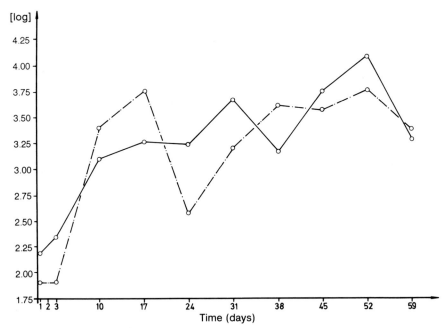

Fig. 4. Counts of coagulase-negative staphylococci/cm^2 forearm skin vs. time (*solid line* = soap first) (from [10])

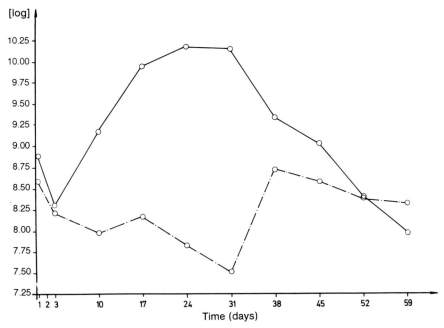

Fig. 5. Counts of propionibacteria/cm² forhead skin vs. time (*solid line* = soap first) (from [10])

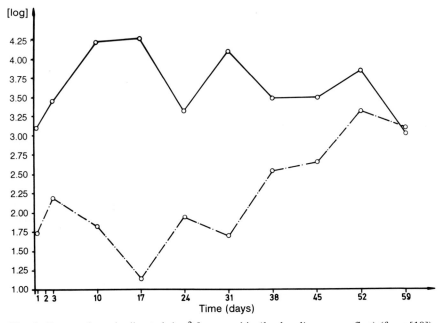

Fig. 6. Counts of propionibacteria/cm² forearm skin (*broken line* = soap first) (from [10])

plasma coagulation test, and biochemical tests using a commercial kit (API STAPH, BioMérieux, Nürtingen, FRG); propionibacteria (Propionibacterium acnes etc.) were identified by Gram staining and the use of appropriate biochemical kits (API 20A, BioMérieux). The results were analyzed using the Wilcoxon tests for paired samples and for independent samples, and the Bravais and Pearson correlation coefficient test. Once in the trial, pH and microbial densities were determined, for each subject, in the period following a washing session, with measurements at 30 minute intervals during a four-hour period.

Under baseline conditions, the pH of the skin was found once again to be in the acid range, with values of between 4.48 and 5.63 on the forehead, and between 4.22 and 5.44 on the forearm. In the subjects who were using soap as the first agent, there was a rise in pH; when these subjects started using the synthetic cleanser, the pH went down again. In the subjects who started washing with the acid pH synthetic cleanser, the skin surface pH remained stable or tended to become more acid yet; when these subjects were crossed over, the pH rose above the baseline values. By the end of Week 2, the pH of those using the synthetic cleanser was significantly lower ($p < 0.01$), and remained at a lower level throughout the study period ($p < 0.05$). The global analysis of all the data shows the skin surface pH to be lower by 0.3 units when the acid pH synthetic cleanser was being used ($p < 0.01$). The analysis of the short-term effects of washing shows a rise in pH, both for synthetic cleanser and for soap; with soap, however, having a much more pronounced effect ($p = 0.01$). As far as the synthetic cleanser is concerned, it is interesting to note that its pH of 5.5 was slightly above the skin pH of the subjects. Any change in pH that had occurred was very largely reversed within two hours (details in the paper by M. Kober).

No definite change in the counts of coagulase-negative staphylococci as a function of the agent used could be established. Only on the forehead was there a significant increase in the population density ($p = 0.05$) when washing with the synthetic cleanser was followed by washing with soap. Propionibacteria (mainly, and numerically in that order, P. acnes and P. granulosum) showed a different pattern: With repeated washing with soap, their counts increased substantially, by about a power of ten; when soap was replaced by the synthetic cleanser, the counts decreased again, in some cases to below the baseline values. In subjects who were using the synthetic cleanser first, there was a significant decrease in the counts of propionibacteria, followed by a significant increase when they started washing with soap. From Week 2 onwards, the foreheads showed significantly higher counts ($p < 0.1$; $p = 0.02$; $p = 0.02$); while on the forearms, significant differences were observed by the end of Week 1 ($p < 0.01$; $p < 0.05$; $p < 0.01$; $p < 0.01$). Overall, with soap, significantly more propionibacteria were found on the forehead and the forearm ($p = 0.02$ and $p = 0.01$, respectively). On the forehead, there was a correlation with skin pH of the densities of coagulase-negative staphylococci and propionibacteria, with propionibacteria showing the better correlation, with correlation coefficients of 0.51 ($p < 0.001$) and 0.56 ($p < 0.001$). On the forearm, correlation was established only for propionibacteria, with a correlation coefficient of 0.24 ($p < 0.05$).

Figures 3 and 4 show the population densities of coagulase-negative staphylococci over time, while Figs. 5 and 6 show the patterns observed for propionibacteria.

When these findings are viewed together, it will be seen that, while the change in skin surface pH following each washing session is rapidly reversed within a few hours, repeated washing with either soap or with acid pH synthetic cleansers will produce long-term changes in skin pH. It should also be noted that different agents can influence different organisms of the resident skin flora for different lengths of time. The counts of propionibacteria on the skin are particularly sensitive to the type of agent used. Since in-vitro studies have shown the specific growth rate of P. acnes to be significantly higher at pH 6 than at pH 5.5, and since no such dependence can be observed in a staphylococcal species (S. aureus) [9], it may be assumed that skin pH has a direct influence on the bacterial flora of the skin – an assumption that would be supported by the correlations between population densities and pH quoted above.

These findings may be of importance for the prevention and treatment of acne vulgaris, a frequent skin disorder, in which washing with synthetic cleansers has been thought to be of benefit [19]. The fact that acid pH synthetic cleansers should affect different skin flora organisms in different degrees is also ecologically interesting, since a drop in the number of propionibacteria is not associated with a general de-germing of the kind observed following the use of disinfectants, which may lead to a temporary overgrowth of pathogenic organisms. Although the results described above suggest that the different biological effect on the skin of washing with (alkaline) soap is chiefly due to the (inevitably high) pH of soap, a further study should be undertaken, using a synthetic cleanser of a chemical composition similar to the one employed in the present study, but adjusted to two different pH levels of 5.5 and 8.5, in order to establish once and for all that what has been observed so far is indeed attributable to pH.

Acknowledgement. We are indebted to Dr. Schadenböck, Mainz, for the synthetic cleanser used in our study.

References

1. Braun-Falco O, Korting HC (1986) Der normale pH-Wert der menschlichen Haut. Hautarzt 37: 126–129
2. Burckhardt W (1964) Methoden zur Untersuchung der Wirkung synthetischer Waschmittel auf die Haut. Dermatologica 129: 37–46
3. Cornbleet T (1933) Self-sterilizing powers of the skin. V. Are they endowed by the surface acid? Arch Dermatol Syph 28: 526–531
4. Foley EJ, Herrmann F, Lee SW (1947) The effects of the pH on the antifungal activity of fatty acids and other agents. Preliminary report. J Invest Dermatol 8: 1–2
5. Freinkel RK, Shen Y (1969) The origin of free fatty acids in sebum. II. Assay of the lipases of the cutaneous bacteria of effects of pH. J Invest Dermatol 53: 422–427

6. Hartmann AA, Röckl H (1979) Vergleichende Untersuchung über den Einfluß von Balneum Hermal Gel zum Duschen auf die aerobe Residentflora der Haut bei einmaliger Anwendung. Ärztl Kosmetol 9: 16–25
7. Heuss E (1892) Die Reaktion des Schweißes beim gesunden Menschen. Monatsh prakt Dermatol 14: 343, 400, 501
8. Holt RJ (1971) Aerobic bacterial counts on human skin after bathing. J Med Microbiol 4: 319–327
9. Korting HC, Bau A, Baldauf P (1987) pH-Abhängigkeit des Wachstumsverhaltens von Staphylococcus aureus und Propionibacterium acnes. Implikationen einer In-vitro-Studie für den optimalen pH-Wert von Hautwaschmitteln. Ärztl Kosmetol 17: 41–53
10. Korting HC, Kober M, Mueller M, Braun-Falco O (1987) Influence of repeated washings with soap and synthetic detergents on pH and resident flora of the skin of forehead and forearm. Results of the cross-over trial in healthy probitioners. Acta Derm Venereol (Stockh) 67: 41–47
11. Marchionini A (1929) Untersuchungen über die Wasserstoffionenkonzentration der Haut. Arch Dermatol Syph 158: 290–333
12. Marchionini A, Hausknecht W (1938) Säuremantel der Haut und Bakterienabwehr. I. Mitteilung. Die regionäre Verschiedenheit der Wasserstoffionenkonzentration der Hautoberfläche. Klin Wochenschr 17: 663–666
13. Marchionini A, Schmidt R (1938) Säuremantel der Haut und Bakterienabwehr. III. Mitteilung. Über die regionäre Verschiedenheit des Bakterienwachstums auf der Hautoberfläche. Klin Wochenschr 17: 773–775
14. Marchionini A, Schmidt R, Kiefer J (1938) Säuremantel der Haut und Bakterienabwehr. II. Mitteilung. Über die regionäre Verschiedenheit der Bakterienabwehr und Desinfektionskraft der Hautoberfläche. Klin Wochenschr 17: 736–739
15. Miescher G (1955) Discussion contribution. Arch Dermatol Syph 200: 53–58
16. Peukert L (1941) Einfluß der Titrationsalkalität von Reinigungsmitteln auf den pH-Wert der menschlichen Haut. Arch Dermatol 181: 417–424
17. Pillsbury DM, Rebell G (1952) The bacterial flora of the skin. Factors influencing the growth of resident and transient organisms. J Invest Dermatol 18: 173–186
18. Pösl H, Schirren CG (1986) Beeinflussung des pH-Wertes der Hautoberfläche durch Seifen, Waschmittel und synthetische Detergentien. Hautarzt 17: 37–40
19. Reichert U, Saint-Leger, G, Schaefer H (1982) Skin surface chemistry and microbial infection. Sem Dermatol 1: 91–99
20. Röckl H, Pascher G (1960) Der Einfluß wasserlöslicher Bestandteile der Hornschicht auf Bakterien. II. Mitteilung. Arch klin exper Dermatol 210: 531–536
21. Röckl H, Spier HB, Pascher G (1957) Der Einfluß wasserlöslicher Bestandteile der Hornschicht auf Bakterien. I. Mitteilung. Arch clin exper Dermatol 205: 420–434
22. Schade, H, Marchionini A (1928) Der Säuremantel der Haut (nach Gaskettenmessung). Klin Wochenschr 7: 12–14
23. Schade H, Marchionini A (1928) Zur physikalischen Chemie der Hautoberfläche. Arch Dermatol Syph 154: 690–716
24. Schirren CG (1955) Does the glass-electrode determine the same pH values on the skin surface as a quinhydrone electrode? J Invest Dermatol 24: 485–488
25. Sharlit H, Scheer M (1923) The hydrogen-ion concentration on the surface of the healthy intact skin. Arch Dermatol Syph 7: 592–598
26. Williamson P, Kligman AM (1965) A new method for the quantitative investigation of cutaneous bacteria. J Invest Dermatol 45: 498–503

In-Vitro Control of the Growth of Important Bacteria of the Resident Skin Flora by Changes in pH

A. Lukacs

Background

Ever since the introduction, by Schade and Marchionini in 1928, of the concept of the skin acid mantle [8], scientists have been debating the relevance of this concept to the bacterial flora of the skin. Pillsbury and Rebell [6] were able to show that a pH of 3.8 is markedly bacteriostatic; while Röckl et al. [7] and Marchionini et al. [5] found a reduction in the counts of Staphylococcus aureus and Staphylococcus albus at pH 5 as compared with pH 7. While not actually deficient in nutrients, the culture medium used was a minimal one. Korting et al. [3] did similar studies using S. aureus and Propionibacterium acnes in trypticase soy broth. The studies were done in buffered solutions, but without additional aeration during bacterial growth. For P. acnes, no oxygen should be added to the gaseous atmosphere; for S. aureus, additional oxygen, while not actually required, might be useful in view of the aerobic conditions on the skin surface. The pH ranges investigated were 5.0–8.0 for S. aureus, and a slightly narrower range of 5.5–7.5 for P. acnes. Colony densities were determined photometrically. Growth was measured in terms of the specific growth rate (number of doublings per hour, or the reciprocal of the time taken for doubling). Figure 1 shows the growth rate of S. aureus plotted against pH. The optimum pH is between 7.0 and 7.5. Figure 2 shows the specific growth rate of P. acnes as a function of pH, with optimum growth at a pH between 6.0 and 6.5. This tallies with the observations of Holland and Cunliffe [2], who, in chemostat experiments, found P. acnes to grow best at pH 6.0. However, there are some inherent weaknesses in the methodology used by Korting et al. [3], which affect the validity of the results:

- A liquid culture medium will sooner or later become depleted in nutrients. Consequently, accurate information can be obtained only for the initial phase of growth. Only little information can be obtained on the plateau phase, i.e. the count that could be attained with constant nutrient supply, since by that time some of the substrate may have been consumed. It would, therefore, be desirable to have the organisms in a steady state.
- The study would also seem to suffer from the fact that the conditions in a shaken or agitated Erlenmeyer flask are not truly representative of the aerobic conditions on the skin surface.

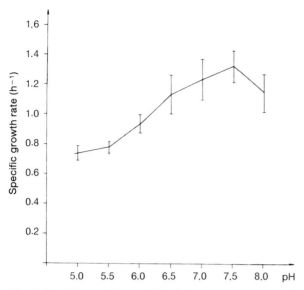

Fig. 1. Specific growth rate of *Staphylococcus aureus* as a function of pH (from [3])

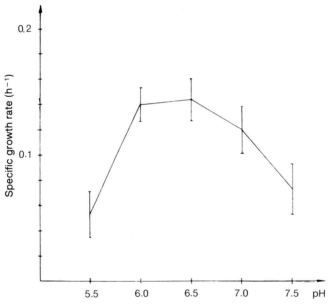

Fig. 2. Specific growth rate of *Propionibacterium acnes* as a function of pH (from [3])

- It is also difficult to have pH control of the buffered solutions. In some experiments, additional titration had to be performed to prevent fluctuations by more than 0.2 units.

Methods

The problems listed above can be obviated by the use of a bioreactor (Fig. 3). This device permits temperature control to within a tenth of a degree; constant stirring speed; a constant gas supply rate (in this study: 0.2 L/min), keeping the oxygen tension at over 90% of the initial value; and constant pH to within 0.1 unit, achieved by the addition of an adjusting agent. The vessel volume is 900 mL, the flow 90 mL/h. The organisms are plated onto blood agar for counting the colony forming units (CFU). The test organism chosen as a result of our own investigations (Korting et al., in preparation) was Staphylococcus epidermidis

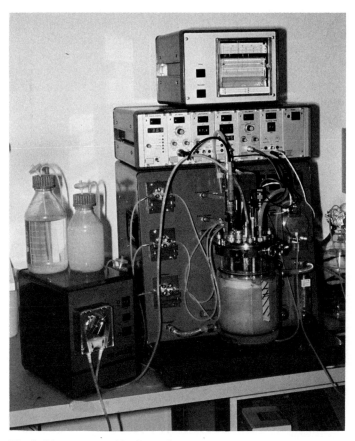

Fig. 3. Bioreactor used in the study

numerically one of the most important organisms of healthy skin. The individual strain carrying the No. 470 represented a recent skin isolate from our clinic. Studies were performed at pH levels of 5.5, 7.0, and 8.5. A trial run was made to find the ranges at which growth would occur. Once the study proper had been started, in order to ensure comparability, no pH changes were effected during the runs, and the pH of the culture solution was adjusted prior to inoculation. Counting was done hourly for the first 12 hours in order to detect delayed growth and rate of growth; and thereafter every 12 hours in order to observe whether a plateau had occurred.

Results

Figure 4 shows the growth of the test strain of S. epidermidis in CFU per mL (log plot) at pH 5.5 during the first 12 hours. The initial lag phase is followed by a phase of exponential growth. A regression line has been drawn to determine the specific growth rate, i.e. the number of doublings per hour. Figure 5 shows the pattern over the entire 8 days of the study. A plateau is reached at 9.2, i.e. at ca. $1.5 \cdot 10^9$ CFU/mL. The trial was repeated, including once again the drawing of a regression line to determine the specific growth rate, and the observation of counts over time.

The same procedure was used at pH 7.0. Again, the test was duplicated. The results were similar to those obtained at pH 5.5, and are described more fully below.

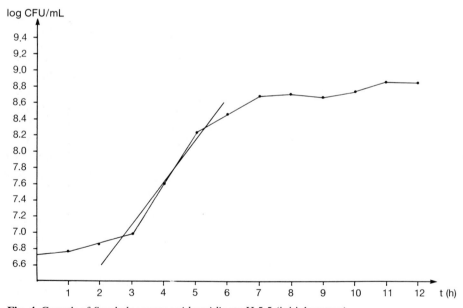

Fig. 4. Growth of *Staphylococcus epidermidis* at pH 5.5 (initial pattern)

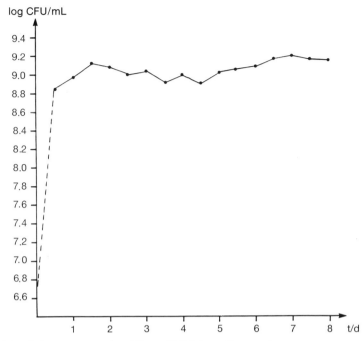

Fig. 5. Growth of *Staphylococcus eperdermidis* at pH 5.5 (overall pattern)

The third pH level chosen was 8.5. At this pH, growth was noticeably delayed, as seen in Figure 6. It took 48 hours to reach the initial count. Also, there is a strikingly low plateau at 8.6, i.e. ca. $0.4 \cdot 10^9$ CFU/mL – one fourth of the numbers at pH 5.5. To illustrate the situation, all the regression lines from the first 12 hours are shown in a diagram (Fig. 7). It will be seen that the results are very reproducible. The best growth is observed at pH 5.5, with only slightly weaker growth at pH 7.0, and a reduction in the number of organisms at the start of the experiments conducted at pH 8.5. Figure 8 once more shows growth at pH 5.5, 7.0, and 8.5, in the form of a bar chart, with the specific growth rate on the ordinate. The broken line bar stands for the later growth phase (between 48 hours and 60 hours after the start of the experiment) at pH 8.5. Again, growth at pH 8.5 is markedly less than at pH 7.0 or even pH 5.5. Figure 9 shows the various plateaux. It will be seen that the number of CFU is highest at pH 5.5, closely followed by the number at pH 7.0 (ca. $1.5 \cdot 10^9$ CFU). The CFU level is lowest at pH 8.5 (ca. $0.4 \cdot 10^9$).

In summary, the studies to date (Korting et al., in preparation) suggest that, at acid pH levels, S. epidermidis shows
- a shorter time from the start of the test to the exponential growth phase;
- subsequent faster growth; and
- a higher ultimate number of CFU.

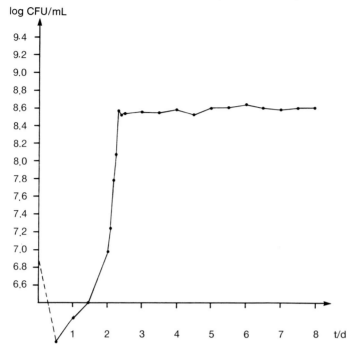

Fig. 6. Growth of *Staphylococcus epidermidis* at pH 8.5

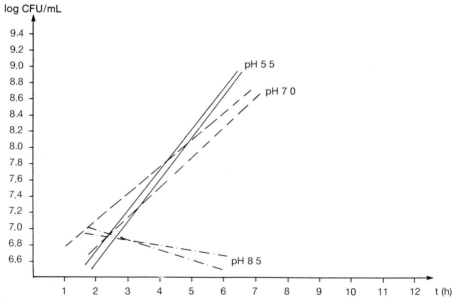

Fig. 7. Regression lines of the first 12 hours

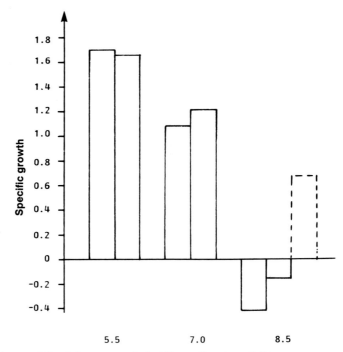

Fig. 8. Specific growth rate of *Staphylococcus epirdimidis* as a function of pH

Discussion

These results may seem surprising. The acid mantle concept might lead one to expect lower numbers and slower growth of organisms at acid pHs. However, since S. epidermidis is a nonpathogenic agent almost always found on the skin, the results, on closer scrutiny, are not all that astonishing. Apart from the situation in intertriginous areas, the pH of the skin is acid [1]. Our investigations have shown that S. epidermidis will, in general, grow better at an acid pH. Thus, what may appear as a contradiction makes perfect sense.

We do not as yet know whether the skin has an inherently acid pH that provides a hospitable environment for S. epidermidis; or whether the organism is attracted by other factors to colonize the skin frequently and in large numbers, and whether, once there, it contributes somehow to the acid reaction of the skin. S. epidermidis, which is nonpathogenic in itself, may also be considered to exert a protective function, in that its presence will prevent overgrowth of the skin by other, pathogenic, bacteria. Also, cross-over studies in healthy volunteers have shown a skin pH difference of only 0.3 units between subjects using an acid pH synthetic cleanser (pH 5.5) and those using an alkaline soap [4]. In the same study, it was found that the counts of S. epidermidis did not differ significantly between the two groups. For other organisms, especially diphtheroids, to be-

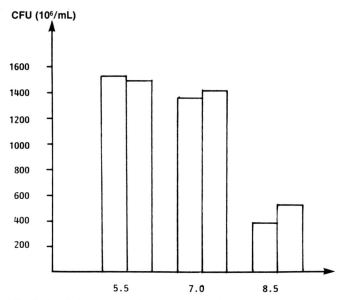

Fig. 9. *Staphylococcus epidermidis* count plateaux as a function of pH

come numerically important on human skin, an alkaline pH level would be required. Thus, to take one of the simplest examples, the microbial pattern in the armpit, with its alkaline pH, is very different from that on exposed glabrous skin.

While, in the study quoted above, the difference in pH was comparatively slight, repeated washing with an acid pH synthetic cleanser was followed by much reduced counts of propionibacteria on the skin. It would, therefore, be interesting to repeat the study with this organism, which has been considered as a major factor in the causation of acne vulgaris (pimples).

Batch culture studies as described above using P. acnes have shown the specific growth rate of this organism to be much more dependent on slightly different pH values in the weakly acid range than was the case with the staphylococcal agent investigated. Preliminary studies using the system described in this paper also seem to suggest this dependency. The design could also be used for a more detailed analysis of the pH dependence of the action of fatty acids, about which there is, as yet, speculation rather than established knowledge.

References

1. Braun-Falco O, Korting HC (1986) Der normale pH-Wert der menschlichen Haut. Hautarzt 37: 126–129
2. Holland KT, Cunliffe WJ, Roberts CD (1978) The role of bacteria in acne vulgaris: A new approach. Clin Exper Dermatol 3: 253–257

3. Korting HC, Bau A, Baldauf P (1987) pH-Abhängigkeit des Wachstumsverhaltens von Staphylococcus aureus und Propionibacterium acnes. Ärzl Kosmetol 17: 41–53
4. Korting HC, Kober M Mueller M, Braun-Falco O (1987) Influence of repeated washings with soap and synthetic detergents on pH and resident flora of the skin of forehead and forearm. Acta Derm Venereol 67: 41–47
5. Marchionini A, Pascher G, Röckl H (1963) Der pH-Wert der Hautoberfläche und seine Bedeutung im Rahmen der Bakterienabwehr. In: Pillsbury DM, Livingood CS (eds) Proceedings of the XIIth Int. Congress of Dermatology. Vol 1, Int. Congresss Scries Nr. 55, Excerpta Medica Foundation, Amsterdam, pp 396–403
6. Pillsbury DM, Rebell G (1952) The bacterial flora of the skin. J Invest Dermatol 18: 173–186
7. Röckl H, Spier HW, Pascher G (1928) Der Einfluß wasserlöslicher Bestandteile der Hornschicht auf Bakterien. Arch Klin Exper Dermatol 205: 420–434
8. Schade H, Marchionini A (1928) Der Säureschutzmantel der Haut. Klin Wochenschr 7: 12–14

Skin Surface Structure

Structure of Human Skin, and Influence of Environmental Factors Such as pH on the Growth of Keratinocytes – Results of Cell Culture Experiments

R. Soehnchen

Physiological Skin pH

Ever since Schade and Marchionini's first description, in 1928 [6], of the acid mantle of the skin, there have been many papers on the pH of the skin surface [4]. Whilst there is no universal agreement on the actual value, the pH of skin would appear to be quite definitely in the acid range. For morphological and anatomical reasons, the detailed in-vitro studies of the relationships between the skin and pH must be confined to the epidermis.

The interactions between epidermal cells and pH may be studied both in vivo, in human epidermis; and in vitro, using cell culture models.

This paper is concerned with some specific biochemical properties of the epidermis with regard to pH, and will also describe studies of cultured human keratinocytes.

Acid and Basic Components of the Epidermis

The human epidermis shows stratified differentiation, with epidermal cell populations in the different strata that are not only morphologically different from each other, but which also display stratum-specific keratin compositions and, hence, specific biochemical features. Keratins provide the intermediate filaments that are typical of epithelial cells; like actin and tubulin, they form the basic scaffolding of cells.

Two-dimensional gel electrophoresis permits the neat separation of cell proteins, with the different molecular weights on the vertical axis, and the differences as a result of isoelectric focusing – i.e. pH – at right angles.

According to Franke et al. [2], epidermal keratins may be classified by their molecular weights, as well as by their isoelectric points in either the acid or the alkaline range.

In the human epidermis, it will be seen that each class of keratin is expressed at a different stage of keratinocyte development, with the alkaline keratins of higher molecular weight occurring chiefly in the upper layers of the epidermis, while the more acid, lower molecular weight classes tend to be expressed in the lower layers.

The relevance of these findings to the physiological protective function of the acid mantle remains to be established, and will undoubtedly be the subject of further studies.

Cultured Epithelial Cells and pH

Cell culturing techniques developed some years ago have made it possible to culture human epithelial cells and to obtain tissue expansion in vitro. This means that scientists are now able to produce large sheets of cells from small epithelial islands. The material thus obtained can then be used, e.g. as a skin substitute in burns patients [7].

These techniques also permit the study, under defined in-vitro conditions, of the proliferation and differentiation characteristics of keratinocytes.

There are two main culturing techniques: Rheinwald and Green's 3T3 cell feeder layer technique [5], with a very complex and rich culture medium and a high expansion factor; and the method described by Eisinger et al. [1], using a simple medium (MEM, L-glutamine, nonessential aminoacids, hydrocortisone, 10% fetal bovine serum) and a defined pH, but producing a much lower expansion factor.

Eisinger et al. found optimum growth to be achieved at pH 5.8–6.0, in submersed cultures at 37 °C in air containing 5% CO_2.

In explant cultures, Karasek [3] found epithelial growth to be maximal at a pH of 7.4, with markedly decreased growth at a more acid or more alkaline pH.

Material and Methods

We used the medium described by Eisinger et al. [1], but at a different, adjusted pH, to perform parallel cultures of human keratinocytes. Whereas in media with a low calcium level, differentiation is suppressed in favour of proliferation, the medium used in our studies permits the cells to express signs of differentiation.

For our investigations, twelve 25 cm^2 culture vessels were seeded with 5×10^6 keratinocytes from the same skin donor (safety margin in removal of melanoma). During the first 4 days, the pH was maintained at 6.0 to permit the attachment of cells capable of proliferation. As a result, constant cell counts in the vessels were not obtained until after the first change of culture medium.

The pH of the medium was adjusted to 5.0, 6.0, and 7.0, using 1 N HCl and 1 N NaOH, respectively. In order to prevent the CO_2 in the incubator atmosphere from producing equilibration, 50 mM Tris buffer (5 mL/100 mL medium) was added to the media. By this means, the pH could be kept reasonably constant. The medium was changed daily, with the addition of fresh medium of adjusted pH at every change.

For the determination of cell counts, trypsin was added to one culture vessel in each pH group, on Days 4, 8, 10, and 14, and individual cell suspensions were produced. Cell counts were made using a Niebauer chamber.

Quantitative pH measurements in the medium were done using a Beckman pH meter (Smith Kline Beckman, Munich, FRG).

Results and Discussion

Proliferation and Differentiation

At pH 6.0, there was a slow and steady increase in the cell count over the observation period. On Day 8 (Fig. 1), the count was ca. 6.5×10^6 cells per vessel. It was noted that, by the time confluency was reached (ca. Days 10–14), proliferation had been arrested by contact inhibition. With continued culturing, only ca. $3-4 \times 10^5$ cells per cm^2 of culture surface area could be seen. The ability to multiply was lost before confluency was obtained. Morphologically, the cells were basal keratinocytes (Fig. 2), with large nuclei and scanty cytoplasm. When viewed from above, they showed the typical pavement-like pattern of confluent cultures, with pale yellow agglomerations of keratinocytes as a sign of incipient differentiation. In some places, multi-layered, stratified structures were observed.

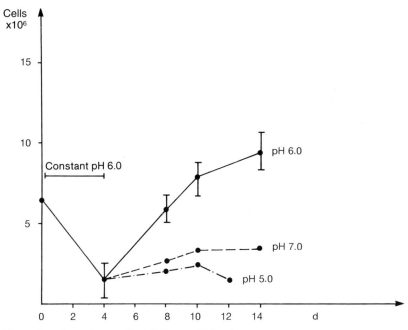

Fig. 1. Keratinocyte growth at different pH levels

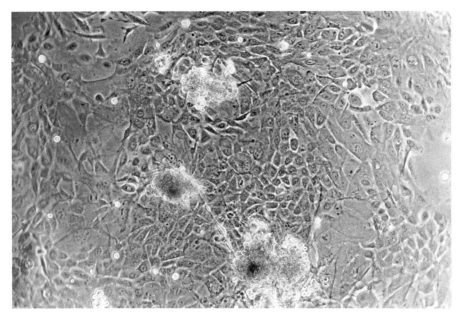

Fig. 2. Keratinocyte culture; pH 6.0; Day 8

Under identical culturing conditions but using a medium of different pH (5.0), a marked reduction in proliferation was seen as early as the 4th day following the change in pH (Day 8 of culturing) (Fig. 1). On Days 10 and 14, there was no significant increase in the cell count, the number being about the same as that of the cells that had attached by Day 4. Thus, at pH 5.0, the cells' proliferative capacity was completely abolished; some cells even died and were found floating in the medium. The large cells, with small nuclei, were found to secrete tiny black granules (Fig. 3). As the culture was continued, all the remaining cells in the medium became detached.

Equally, a neutral pH of 7.0 was suboptimal for keratinocyte growth. Following the pH change, only low cell counts were observed after 8 and 10 days of culturing, and no further proliferative tendency was noted between that stage and Day 14. By then, there remained only some clusters of keratinocytes on the bottom of the culture vessels; unlike cells grown under optimal conditions, the material at pH 7.0 showed no tendency towards confluent growth. Proliferation was much slower; however, the cells did not die, neither did they secrete black granules into the medium. Most strikingly, at pH 7.0, fibroblast growth was markedly increased: By Day 14, there were sometimes large areas of proliferating fibroblasts among the keratinocyte clusters, which were in danger of being overgrown by the fibroblasts.

The morphological pattern at pH 7.0 was marked by comparatively small nuclei with much cytoplasm, i.e. the typical pattern of non-proliferating cells. The boundaries of the cell colonies were formed by cell bodies that appeared to

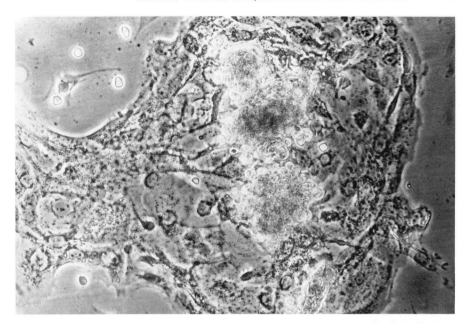

Fig. 3. Keratinocyte culture; pH 5.0; Day 8

trail off peripherally. The situation at pH 7.0 seems to differ from that at pH 6.0 in that, at the more neutral pH, differentiation was initiated, without the proliferative potential of the cells being exhausted.

Efficiency of Colony Formation

In addition to proliferation and differentiation, human epithelial cell colony formation – as a measure of the dividing capacity of the individual keratinocytes – may be determined in vitro.

In such studies, care should be taken to ensure that cells are seeded at comparatively low densities. Following an initial inoculum of 5×10^5 cells per 60 mm Petri dish, much better colony formation was seen, at 3 weeks, in media kept at pH 6.0 as compared with more acidic or more alkaline levels (Fig. 4).

The cells observed were comparatively small, with large nuclei and little cytoplasm, which indicates that they have a high proliferation potential.

The results were markedly less favourable when the pH was kept between 5.8 and 6.7. Under these conditions, colony formation was much reduced, and the cells showed no morphological evidence of any major proliferation potential.

At pH 5.8, the ability to form colonies was particularly compromised. At that level, only tiny colonies were found after 3 weeks' culturing. Optimum growth was seen at pH 6.0, i.e. only 0.2 units above the particularly adverse level.

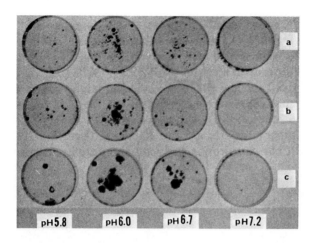

Fig. 4. Colony formation at different pH levels

Secretion of Acidic Substances by Epithelial Cells

The medium used for keratinocyte cultures contains phenol red, which provides a rough indication of pH.

A colour change to yellow-red is indicative of an acid pH, while a purple discoloration of the medium indicates an alkaline pH. This indicator provides a ready qualitative means of detecting pH changes in the medium. As a rule, the keratinocyte culture medium is changed every 3 days. It was noted that, as time went by, the cultures, which had originally been purple, tended to become increasingly yellowish-red.

At the first change of medium, initial cultures had a purple medium. This was probably due to the fact that only a small proportion of the cells are metabolically active by that stage. Older, confluent cultures, on the other hand, have many actively growing cells. These cultures tended to show increasing yellowing of the medium, which suggests secretion of acidic substances into the medium. In fibroblasts, this colour change was not found even after confluency had been reached.

When this qualitative observation was studied quantitatively, with sampling of the unbuffered medium and determination in the pH meter, it was found that, with increasing duration of the culture, the pH would become increasingly acid (Fig. 5).

In newly seeded cultures, pH values of about 6.8 were found two days after the introduction of fresh medium. In actively proliferating cultures, the level noticeably dropped into the acid range, falling steadily from Days 8–10 onwards. On Day 14, with complete confluency, the pH values found were around 6.0. No further drop was found as the culture continued.

Unlike fibroblasts, keratinocytes in vitro appear to secrete acid metabolic products into the medium; equally, optimum cell growth requires an acid milieu.

It is conceivable that in vivo this mechanism is involved in the homeostasis of the acid mantle of the skin.

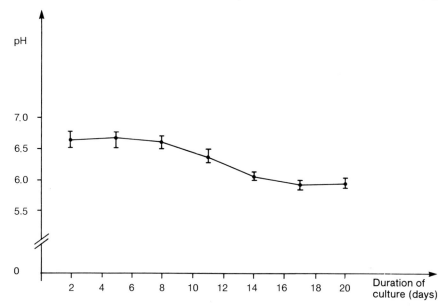

Fig. 5. Culture medium pH

References

1. Eisinger M, Lee JS, Hefton JM, Darzynkiewicz Z, Chiao J, de Harven E (1979) Human epidermal cell cultures: growth and differentiation in absence of dermal components or medium supplements. Proc Natl Acad Sci (Washington) 76: 5340–5344
2. Franke WW, Schmid E, Schiller DL, Winter S, Jarasch ED, Moll R, Denk H, Jackson BW, Illmensee K (1982) Differentiation-related pattern of expression of proteins of intermediate size filaments in tissues and cultured cells. Cold Spring Harbor Symp Quant Biol 46: 431–453
3. Karasek M (1966) In vitro culture of human skin ephithelial cells. J Invest Dermatol 47: 533–540
4. Braun-Falco O, Korting HC (1986) Der normale pH-Wert der menschlichen Haut. Hautarzt 37: 126–129
5. Rheinwald J, Green H (1975) Serial cultivation of strains of human epidermal keratinocytes: formation of colonies from single cells. Cell 6: 331–344
6. Schade H, Marchionini A (1928) Der Säuremantel der Haut. Klin Wochenschr 7: 12–14
7. Soehnchen R, Braun-Falco O (1988) Epitheltransplantation mit kultivierten Keratinozyten. Hautarzt 39: 701–707

Skin Roughness – Measuring Methods and Dependence on Washing Procedure

D. Vieluf

Background

In dermatological research, macroscopic and microscopic investigations of the skin surface have been undertaken for a long time. Table 1 lists the methods used.

Table 1. Methods for the visualization and assessment of skin topography

- Clinical examination
- Surface microscopy
- Skin surface photography
- SEM studies of skin or epidermal biopsy specimens
- Skin surface biopsy (SSB) assessment using light, stereo, or scanning electron microscopy
- Replication procedures (assessment by photography, light microscopy, or SEM)
- Profilometry

The clinical examination of the skin surface permits only a qualitative assessment by the investigator. Special optical aids have been developed which permit in-situ microscopic studies of the skin's topography, with up to 50-fold magnification. This so-called surface microscopy usually offers the additional facility of taking photographs of the skin surface [8, 16, 59]. While these microscopic techniques provide more information than could be obtained from simple macroscopic clinical examination, they only permit a subjective and purely qualitative assessment. Macrophotography of the skin can be done at low magnification only, and does not really give an idea of the three-dimensional nature of the topography [11, 42].

Taking epidermal or full-thickness skin biopsy specimens and examining them with SEM (14, 20, 28, 41, 48, 49] does not permit monitoring the course of a disorder or the effect of treatment. The technique also suffers from the problem of fixation artefacts that may distort the surface texture.

Skin surface biopsy (SSB) involves the brief application of a liquid adhesive to the skin, followed by the stripping of the stratum corneum or the superficial epidermis, with assessment of the biopsies by light, stereo, or scanning electron microscopy [1, 4, 9, 14, 18, 19, 34, 37, 39, 50, 51, 57, 61, 67]. SSB provides information on such parameters as intraepidermal cohesion or changes in the corneocytes (e. g. in various skin disorders; as a function of age; or as a result of topical dermatological therapy). However, it will not give quantifiable and objective information on the skin surface.

The replication procedures, with assessment by light microscopy or SEM (as well as photography), do not have the disadvantages discussed above; however, they, too, rely upon descriptive criteria that will produce a qualitative statement which, more often than not, cannot be substantiated [3, 7, 12, 13, 15, 17, 27, 33, 36, 53, 55, 56, 61, 65].

In order to obtain reproducible values that can be used for a more detailed objective characterization of the morphology of the skin's surface, profilometry has been introduced into dermatological research as a comparatively straightforward method of measurement that yields parameters of a kind used worldwide in industrial engineering and defined in international ISO (International Organization for Standardization) and German DIN (Deutsche Industrie-Norm) standards [2, 6, 23, 24, 26, 35, 38].

Several researchers are now using this method in dermatology, especially to assess the effects of cosmetics or drugs on the skin surface [5, 44, 45, 46, 54].

Profilometry provides quantitative information in the form of roughness parameters such as the arithmetical mean deviation of the profile R_a and the mean depth of roughness R_{ZDIN}, for which there are ISO and DIN standards (cf. above). Other parameters include the maximum height of the profile R_y or maximum depth of roughness R_{max}, and R_{ZISO} (cf. Table 2). While these parameters reflect deviations in a vertical direction, profilometry can, in principle, also be used to measure deviations in a horizontal direction (e. g. by detecting the mean spacing of profile irregularities, and periodicities), and to obtain at least some information on the so-called shape factor [22]. However, these aspects are not routinely considered in dermatological research. In general, profilometry provides information on surface roughness, not only of engineering materials and components, but also of the human skin.

Methods for the Study of Skin Roughness

Frictional Methods

Since the laws of friction apply to the skin as they do to any other surface, the so-called coefficient of friction of the skin can be determined by using the formula $F = \mu \cdot L$, where F is the frictional force, L is the load or force normal to the surface, and μ is the coefficient of friction, which provides direct information on skin smoothness. Skin friction studies are done using a probe of defined shape which is moved at a constant speed over the surface of interest; equally, a modified rotating viscometer may be used [10, 21, 25, 43, 52, 66].

Table 2. Surface roughness parameters (from ISO Standard 4287 and DIN Standards 4768 and 4762)

Parameter		Definition	
Parameter	Symbol		
Arithmetical mean deviation of the profile	R_a	$R_a = \dfrac{1}{I_m} \times \displaystyle\int_{x=0}^{x=I_m} \|y\|\, dx$	
		The arithmetical mean of the absolute values of the profile departures within the sampling length l, after filtering of shape departures and the coarser elements of waviness	
Mean depth of roughness	R_{ZDIN}	$R_Z = \dfrac{1}{5}(Z_1 + Z_2 + Z_3 + Z_4 + Z_5)$	
		The arithmetical mean of the depths of roughness of five adjacent sampling lengths of equal length, of the profile filtered in accordance with DIN 4768 Sheet 1 (= R_{y5} in the ISO system)	
Maximum height of the profile (ISO)	R_y	The distance between the line of profile peaks and the line of the profile valleys within the sampling length	
Maximum depth of roughness (DIN)	R_{max}	Maximum depth of roughness Z_i within the evaluation length l_m found in the measurement of R_{ZDIN}, of the profile filtered in accordance with DIN 4768 Sheet 1 (= $R_{y\,max}$ in the ISO system)	
Ten point height of irregularities	R_{ZISO}	$R_{ZISO} = \dfrac{1}{5} \times \left(\displaystyle\sum_{i=1}^{5} Y_{pi} + \sum_{i=1}^{5} Y_{vi} \right)$	
		The average value of the absolute values of the heights of five highest profile peaks and the depths of five deepest profile valleys within the sampling length	

Light Optical Methods

Reflectance Measurements

This method is based upon the fact that a dye applied to the skin will be adsorbed differently to the skin surface as a function of the various features of the skin's topography, producing different staining intensities. The difference in reflectance, measured at 620 nm, between unstained and stained skin provides a direct measure of skin roughness [58, 64].

Table 3. Methods for the study of skin roughness

- Frictional methods
- Light optical methods
-   – Reflectance methods (including densitometry)
-   – Light profilometry
- Acoustical methods
- Contact (stylus) profilometry

Densitometry

In this technique, enlarged macrophotographic negatives of the skin surface are scanned in a densitometer and compared with a defined grey scale. Differences in contrast can thus be quantified and recorded. The total line length traced by the pen over a standard chart length of 15 cm is measured to provide quantification of the roughness of the skin [40].

Light Profilometry

This method involves the projection onto the skin of a line of light through a slit, and photographing this line at an angle of 45°. The ratio of the developed length of the light profile K to a straight sampling length line S drawn from one end of the profile to the other is a measure of surface roughness ($R = K/S$) [60].

Acoustical Methods

In this method, a sled is moved across the skin. The noise produced by this movement is picked up by a microphone on the sled, and processed. The roughness parameter measured is the so-called noise intensity [63].

Contact (Stylus) Profilometry

Profilometry with a scanning probe permits the description of the skin's condition at the time of investigation and provides a permanent record of the sample. First, a replica (negative) of the area to be measured must be produced. Replication materials must comply with certain requirements. They must be
- harmless
- easy to mix
- work at body temperature
- have reasonably short curing times
- reproduce skin details faithfully, and
- have good dimensional accuracy.

There are dental impression materials that meet these requirements and are known to be hypoallergenic and to have a low irritancy potential. Silicones and zinc oxide-eugenol pastes are among the substances that have been successfully used. Whereas the replicas produced by the techniques mentioned earlier [3, 7, 12, 13, 15, 17, 27, 33, 36, 53, 55, 56, 61, 65] are assessed with SEM, contact profilometry relies upon the mechanical scanning of the replicas. A microprobe consisting of a stylus with a thin diamond tip with a defined cone angle of 60° and a tip radius of 5 m is moved at constant speed and with very little friction (load exerted by the stylus tip 0.8 mN) over the negative. The stylus has a Teflon skid to protect the surface traversed.

This Teflon skid also ensures even scanning without any sudden jolts. The motor advances the stylus along a straight line over any given length on the surface to be measured, with the diamond tip probing the surface irregularities. The displacement of the stylus is converted by an inductive transducer into electrical signals and potentials, of amplitudes that are proportional to the deflections of the stylus. The signals thus produced are amplified in a carrier frequency amplifier, and digitized in an analog-digital converter. A microprocessor is used to compute immediately the various surface parameters (according to ISO and DIN standards); the values obtained are then read from an alphanumeric display. At the same time, the equipment gives a graphic output of the surface profile, and logs the data. Contact profilometry has been used in metallurgy to detect surface irregularities of between 0.01 to 1000 μm.

Earlier studies had shown that most skin areas – including the flexor aspect of the forearm, and the forehead – are very finely textured and that, consequently, the error may be assumed to be negligible [22, 24, 35]. The direction of scan on the forearm flexor aspect and on the forehead must be relative to the major skin creases, which are usually normal to the body axis.

This technique constitutes a fairly straightforward means of obtaining reproducible data; five runs along each scan (a total of 6 scans, arranged radially from a central point, at intervals of 30°) will produce sufficiently accurate roughness data. As may be expected, there is very great variation between different skin sites in one and the same subject. Also, there may be much individual variation of the roughness of identical skin areas within the same age group [22, 23]. With increasing age, the skin tends to get rougher in its vertical pattern, as well as coarser in texture. Children have the smoothest vertical transverse profiles, as well as the most finely textured skin. Adult males have greater vertical roughness in almost all skin areas than do females. On average, the roughest sites are the skin over the kneecap, the armpit, and the periumbilical region; while the extensor aspect of the leg (pretibial area), the forehead, and the calf tend to be smoothest [22].

Apart from flexion and extension, the function of the skin will affect skin roughness. Functional aspects play a major rôle in the texture of the skin profile. With increasing age, the skin tends to develop more areas that show a certain lay (a prevailing texture of transverse or longitudinal grooves); also, the lay of any one skin area tends to become more pronounced. On the other hand, the number of skin grooves per unit area tends to decrease.

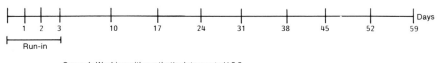

Fig. 1. Influence of different synthetic detergent skin cleansers on skin roughness, TEWL, and skin surface pH. Study design

As a result, when studying the effect of external substances, a comparison should be made at the same site, to see how the parameters mentioned above evolve over time.

Contact profilometry has the disadvantage of producing mechanical filtering of the profile as the surface is scanned by the stylus moving on its skid. Also, because of the shape of the stylus, the vertical dimension of the skin grooves (which, as a rule, are deep, V-shaped structures) may be distorted. There is also the problem of the reduction to a merely two-dimensional graph of the three-dimensional structures of the skin, with consequent loss of information content.

Use of Profilometry in Studies Involving the Use of Skin Cleansing Agents by Healthy Subjects

Study Design

For the study of the effect of different synthetic detergent skin cleansing preparations on skin roughness as well as on transepidermal water loss (TEWL) and skin pH, use can be made of a study design described in a previous paper [31], with the two test substances being used consecutively, in a randomized blind trial. One group of healthy volunteers are instructed to use one of the preparations for a period of four weeks, to clean the skin of the forehead (midline) and the flexor aspect of the forearm distal to the antecubital fossa, mornings and evenings, for 60 seconds each time; with a cross-over to the other preparation, which will then be used in the same way for the next four weeks. The test parameters are measured at the start of the trial, and thereafter at seven day intervals, in the period between the morning and evening washing sessions (not less than 4 hours after the latest use of the cleanser) (cf. Fig. 1).

For profilometry, replicas of the sites to be measured are made using Silasoft N (low viscosity silicone elastomer precision impression material) and its catalyst paste (Detax, Karlsruhe), with a mixing time of 30 sec, working time from the start of mixing of 75 sec, and a curing time of 225 sec (Fig. 2). A Hommel-

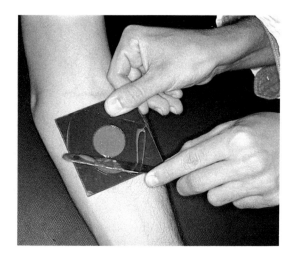

Fig. 2. Replication technique. Use of Silasoft N and catalyst paste (Detax, Karlsruhe) to obtain a skin replica

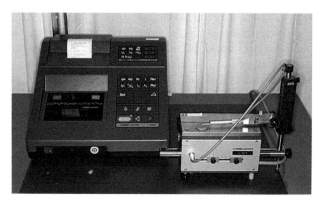

Fig. 3. Hommel-Tester T 2000 profilometer (Hommel-Werke, Villingen-Schwenningen)

Tester T2000 profilometer (Hommel-Werke, Villingen-Schwenningen) (Fig. 3) is used to scan each replica (30 mm diameter) radially, over a half circle, in six directions at 30° intervals (Fig. 4) to obtain and compute the surface parameters (arithmetical mean deviation of the profile R_a, mean depth of roughness R_{ZDIN}, maximum height of the profile R y or maximum depth of roughness R_{max}, and ten point height of irregularities R_{ZISO}) laid down in the standards. Figure 5 shows a typical skin surface profile (along one scan).

After taking the replica for profilometry, other studies are made where required. TEWL is measured using the Servo-Med EP 1 evaporimeter (Servo Med AB, Vällingby, Sweden) (Fig. 6). Readings are taken 30 seconds after the application of the probe to the skin. The ambient temperature is kept at 19°C. Before the measurements are made, subjects are made to rest supine for an adaptation period of 30 minutes. Details of the techniques employed for measur-

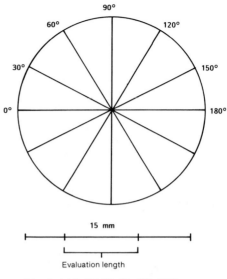

Fig. 4. Scanning a replica with a profilometer

6 lengths (at 0°, 30°, 60°, 90°, 120°, 150°)
each scanned 5 times

ing TEWL and skin surface pH are given elsewhere in this monograph [68] by H. Zienicke, whose studies were conducted in parallel with mine.

If the study design so requires, skin surface pH is measured as a final step, using the Ingold flat glass electrode (403-F7 glass electrode, Ingold-Meßtechnik, Steinbach) connected to a precision pH meter (pH 521, WTW, Weilheim). Every measurement is made three times, using standard methods, and the mean of the measurements is calculated. Studies of this kind have been used in postgraduate research done at Munich University Hospital, and the main results obtained have been published in the literature [29, 30]. The two theses have been concerned with the influence of the pH of a given synthetic cleanser formulation on the bacterial flora and the pH of the skin surface.

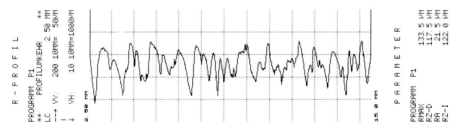

Fig. 5. Typical profilogram obtained from one scan (contact stylus profilometry)

124   D. Vieluf

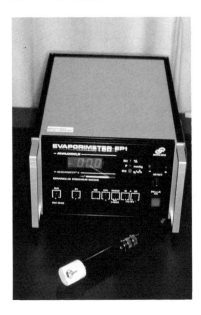

Fig. 6. EP 1 evaporimeter (Servo Med AB, Vällingby, Sweden)

Two liquid synthetic detergent cleansers of pH 5.5 and 8.5, respectively, were used. The former was a commercially available preparation (Sebamed flüssig, Sebapharma, Boppard), the latter had the same chemical composition but had been made alkaline by the addition of NaOH. The two agents were used in 10 healthy subjects (male and female young adults) (cf. [32]).

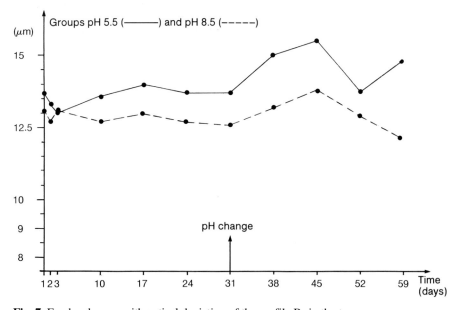

Fig. 7. Forehead mean arithmetical deviation of the profile R_a in the two groups

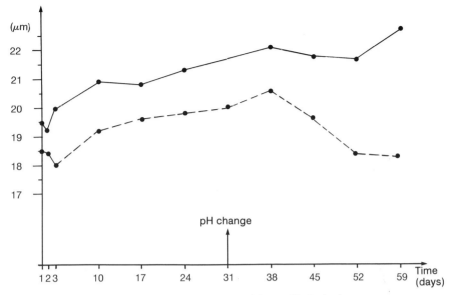

Fig. 8. Left forearm mean arithmetical deviation of the profile R_a in the two groups

Results

Figures 7 and 8 show the arithmetical mean deviation of the profile Ra of the forehead and the forearm vs. time. It is important to note that, when a liquid synthetic detergent cleanser was used regularly twice daily, there was an increase in skin roughness in the short term, which tended to decline as the use of the preparation continued. Following the change to the other preparation used in the trial, there was once again an initial increase in roughness; this pattern was observed regardless of whether the cross-over was from the acidic to the alkaline cleanser or vice versa. While, in certain cases, there is a suggestion that skin roughness may be related to the pH of the synthetic cleanser used, the overall response in terms of R_a did not show any significant difference between the two agents. This tallies with what has been found for TEWL [68]. As far as skin pH was concerned, this study bears out the earlier findings [31] that the repeated use of acidic or alkaline synthetic detergent cleansers will have a sustained effect on skin pH.

Discussion

From the data shown it may be concluded that, contrary to Tronnier's postulate [63], the irritancy potential of a skin cleanser is not a priori a function of cleanser pH. While Nissen and Kreysel's studies [47] would appear to confirm Tronnier's hypothesis, it should be borne in mind that, unlike this present study, their investigation was done using skin cleansers that differed not only in pH but also in their chemical composition.

Quite generally, our experience with profilometry at Munich University Hospital suggests that this method is useful in cosmetological research since it can provide valuable information on the risk potential of substances, including skin cleansers. In future, profilometric comparisons should be done in the course of post-marketing product improvement, in order to find an optimally tolerated formulation. In order to get full benefit from profilometry, the data obtained should provide information on the specific response patterns of healthy subjects of different skin type, age, sex, and – possibly – occupation or lifestyle, to ensure that the test population used is truly representative of the population at large or of the specific target group at which the preparation concerned is aimed (e.g. subjects with sensitive skin etc.).

References

1. Agache P, Maircy J, Boyer JP (1972) Le stripping du stratum corneum au cyanoacrylate. Intérêt en physiologie et en pathologie cutanées. J Med Lyon 53: 1017–1022
2. Barbenel JC, Ferguson J (1980) Skin surface patterns and the directional mechanical properties of the dermis. In: Proceedings of the International Symposium on Bioengineering and the Skin. Cardiff/UK 83–92
3. Berenstein EO, Jones CB (1969) Skin replication procedure for the scanning electron microscope. Science 166: 252–253
4. Chinn HD, Dobson RL (1964) The topographic anatomy of human skin. Arch Dermatol 89: 267–273
5. Cook TH (1980) Profilometry of skin, a useful tool for substantiation of cosmetic efficiency. J Soc Cosmet Chem 31: 339–359
6. Cook TH, Craft TJ, Brurelle RL, Norris F, Griffin WA (1982) Quantification of the skin's topography by skin profilometry. Int J Cosmet Sci 4: 195–205
7. Cseplák G, Martou T (1967) Neue Verfahren zur Dokumentation der Oberfläche gesunder und kranker Haut. Arch Klin Exper Dermatol 228: 414–420
8. Cunliffe WJ, Forester RA, Williams M (1974) A surface microscope for clinical and laboratory use. Brit J Dermatol 90: 619–622
9. Dawber RPR, Marks R, Swift JA (1972) Scanning electron microscopy of the stratum corneum. Brit J Dermatol 86: 272–281
10. El-Shimi AF (1977) In vivo skin friction measurements. J Soc Cosmet Chem 28: 37–51
11. Epstein E (1977) Fast reliable photography for the dermatologist. Int J Dermatol 16: 134–142
12. Facq JM, Kirk D, Rebell G (1964) A simple replica for observation of human skin. J Soc Cosmet Chem 15: 87–98
13. Forck G, Pfantsch M, Fromme HC, Wichelmann F, Tegtbauer C (1972) Zur rasterelektronenmikroskopischen Darstellung der Hautoberfläche mittels Abdruckverfahren. Arch Dermatol Forsch 244: 92–94
14. Franchimont C (1980) The stratum corneum xerotic from aging and photochemotherapy (PUVA). Am J Dermatopathol 2: 295–304
15. Garber CA, Nightingale CT (1976) Characterizing cosmetic effects and skin morphology by scanning electron microscopy. J Soc Cosmet Chem 27: 509–531

16. Goldman L, Younker W (1947) Studies in microscopy of the surface of skin: Preliminary report of techniques. J Invest Dermatol 9: 11
17. Goldman L, Vahl J, Rockwell RJ, Meyer R, Franzen M, Owens P, Hyatt S (1969) Replica microscopy and scanning electron microscopy of laser impacts on the skin. J Invest Dermatol 52: 18–24
18. Goldschmidt H, Kligman AM (1967) Exfoliative cytology of human horny layer. Arch Dermatol 96: 572–576
19. Goldschmidt H, Thew MA (1972) Exfoliative cytology of psoriasis and other common dermatoses. Arch Dermatol 106: 476–483
20. Hashimoto K, Kanzaki T (1975) Surface ultrastructure of human skin. Acta Derm Venereol (Stockh) 55: 413–430
21. Highley DR, Coomey M, Den Beste M, Wolfram LJ (1971) Frictional properties of skin. J Invest Dermatol 69: 303–305
22. Hoestermann U (1986) Rauhigkeitsbestimmungen an menschlicher Haut mit Hilfe des Verfahrens der Profilometrie nach dem Tastschnittprinzip. Thesis, Munich University
23. Hoppe U (1979) Topologie der Hautoberfläche. J Soc Cosmet Chem 30: 213–239
24. Hoppe U, Luderstädt R, Sauermann G (1986) Quantitative Analyse der Hautoberfläche mit Hilfe der digitalen Signalverarbeitung. Ärztl Kosmetol 16: 13–37
25. Jordan R, Streckert G (1981) Beeinflussung der Glätte der Haut durch Baden. Ärztl Kosmetol 11: 260–266
26. Kadner H, Biesold C (1971) Zur Technik der Rauhigkeitsmessung der Hautoberfläche mit dem Perth-O-Meter. Dermatol Monatsschr 157: 758–759
27. Kampik E (1985) Die Struktur der menschlichen Hautoberfläche in verschiedenen Altersstufen – rasterelektronenmikroskopische Untersuchung mit Hilfe der Replica-Methode. Thesis, Munich University
28. Kligman AM, Lavker RM (1982) Some aspects of dry skin and its treatment. In: Kligman AM (Ed), Safety and efficacy of topical drugs and cosmetics. JJ Leyden, New York, London
29. Korting HC, Greiner K, Hübner K, Hamm G (in press) Influence of repeated washings with synthetic detergent preparations of pH 5.5 and 8.5 on the resident flora of the skin of forehead and forearm. Results of a cross-over trial in healthy volunteers. J Soc Cosm Chem
30. Korting HC, Hübner K, Greiner K, Hamm G (in press) Differences in the skin surface pH and bacterial microflora due to the long-term application of synthetic detergent preparations of pH 5.5 and 7.0. Results of a cross-over trial in healthy volunteers. Acta Derm Venereol (Stockh)
31. Korting HC, Kober M, Mueller M, Braun-Falco O (1987) Influence of repeated washings with soap and synthetic detergents on pH and resident flora of the skin of forehead and forearm. Results of a cross-over trial in healthy probitioners. Acta Derm Venereol (Stockh) 67: 41–47
32. Korting HC, Megele M, Mehringer L, Vieluf D, Zienicke H, Hamm G (in preparation) Influence of repeated washings with an acid and an alkaline synthetic detergent preparation of identical chemical composition on pH, roughness and transepidermal water loss of forehead and forearm. Acta Derm Venereol (Stockh)
33. Kuokkanen K (1972) Replica reflection of normal skin and of skin with disturbed keratinization. Acta Derm Venereol (Stockh) 52: 205–210
34. Lachapelle JM, Gouverneur JC, Boulet M, Tennstedt DA (1977) A modified technique (using polyester tape) of skin surface biopsy. Brit J Dermatol 97: 49–52
35. Makki S, Barbenel JC, Agache P (1979) A quantitative method for the assessment of the microtopography of human skin. Acta Derm Venereol (Stockh) 59: 285–291
36. Marks R (1978) Techniques for the evaluation of emollients and keratolytics. J Soc Cosmet Chem 29: 433–440
37. Marks R, Dawber RPR (1971) Skin surface biopsy: an improved technique for the examination of the horny layer. Brit J Dermatol 84: 117–123
38. Marks R, Pearse AD (1975) Surfometry – a method of evaluating the internal structure of the stratum corneum. Brit J Dermatol 92: 651–657

39. Marks R, Saylan T (1972) The surface structure of the stratum corneum. Acta Derm Venereol (Stockh) 52: 119–124
40. Marshall RJ, Marks R (1983) Assessment of skin surface by scanning densitometry of macrophotographs. Clin Exper Dermatol 8: 121–127
41. Menton DN, Eisen AZ (1971) Structural organization of the stratum corneum in certain scaling disorders of the skin. J Invest Dermatol 57: 295–307
42. Moynahan EJ, Engel CE (1962) Photomacrography of the normal skin. Med Biol Illus 12: 72–82
43. Naylor PFD (1955) The skin surface and friction. Brit J Dermatol 67: 239–248
44. Nichols S, King CS, Marks R (1978) Short term effects of emollients and bathoil on the stratum corneum. J Soc Cosmet Chem 29: 617–624
45. Nissen HP, Biltz H, Kreysel HW (1986) Hautrauhigkeitsmessung zur Beurteilung der therapeutischen Wirksamkeit topischer Glucorticoide. Zeitschr Hautkr (Suppl 2) 130–135
46. Nissen HP, Biltz H, Kreysel HW (1988) Profilometrie, eine Methode zur Beurteilung der therapeutischen Wirksamkeit von Kamillosan-Salbe,. Zeitschr Hautkr 63: 184–190
47. Nissen HP, Kreysel HW (1985) Flüssige Waschsyndets verschiedener pH-Wert-Einstellungen. Vergleichende Untersuchungen. Ärztl Kosmetol 15: 304–313
48. Orfanos C, Christenhusz R, Mahrle G (1969) Die normale und psoriatische Hautoberfläche. Vergleichende Beobachtungen mit dem Raster-Elektronenmikroskop. Arch Klin Exper Dermatol 235: 284–294
49. Papa CM, Farber B (1971) Direct scanning electron microscopy of human skin. Arch Dermatol 104: 262–270
50. Piérard-Franchimont C, Piérard GE (1985) Skin surface stripping in diagnosing and monitoring inflammatory, xerotic, and neoplastic diseases. Pediatr Dermatol 2: 180–184
51. Piérard-Franchimont C, Piérard GE (1987) Assessment of aging and actinic damages by cyanoacrylate skin surface stripping. Am J Dermatopathol 9: 500–509
52. Prall JK (1973) Instrumental evaluation of the effects of cosmetic products on skin surfaces with particular references to smoothness. J Soc Cosmet Chem 24: 693–699
53. Ryan RL, Hing SAO, Theiler RF (1983) A replica technique for the evaluation of human skin by scanning electron microscopy. J Cutan Pathol 10: 262–276
54. Salfeld K, Gebhardt K (1973) Vergleichende Untersuchungen zur Wirkungsweise verschiedener "Verjüngungcremes" auf die alternde Haut. Ärztl Kosmetol 3: 108–111
55. Sampson J (1961) A method of replicating dry and moist surfaces for examination by light microscopy. Nature 191: 932–933
56. Sarkany J (1962) A method for studying the microtopography of the skin. Brit J Dermatol 74: 254–259
57. Schellander FA, Headington JT (1974) The stratum corneum – some structural and functional correlates. Brit J Dermatol 91: 507–515
58. Schneider W, Tronnier H, Bussius H (1959) Weitere Untersuchungen an Hautschutzsalben mit einer neuen Methodik. Hautarzt 10: 205–208
59. Siebentritt CR (1949) An apparatus for the examination and photography of the cutaneous surface and skin microtopography. J Invest Dermatol 13: 281–288
60. Szakall A, Stüpel H (1957) Die Wirkung von Waschmitteln auf die Haut. Hüthig Verlag, Heidelberg, 99
61. Tring FC (1974) Surface microtopography of normal human skin. Arch Dermatol 109: 223
62. Tronnier H (1960) Zur Prüfung des Effekts von Rasierhilfsmitteln. Ästhet Med 9: 241–246
63. Tronnier H (1985) Seifen und Syndets in der Hautpflege und -therapie. Ärztl Kosmetol 15: 19–30
64. Tronnier H, Eisbacher T (1970) Über eine neue Methode zur Messung der Rauhigkeit der Haut. Berufsdermatosen 18: 89–95
65. Wagner G, Goltz RW (1979) Human cutaneous topography. Cutis 23: 830–842
66. Weinstein S (1978) New methods for the in-vivo-assessment of skin smoothness and skin softness. J Soc Cosmet Chem 29: 99–115

67. Wolf J (1940) Über die Herstellung mikroskopischer Präparate der Oberflächen verschiedener Objekte mit Hilfe der Adhäsionsmethode. Z wiss Mikroskopie 56: 181–201
68. Zienicke H (1990) Hautfeuchtigkeit (Transepidermaler Wasserverlust) – Meßmethoden und Abhängigkeit von Waschverfahren. In: Braun-Falco O, Korting HC (Eds) Hautreinigung mit Syndets. Springer Verlag
68a Zienicke H (1992) Skin hydration (transepidermal water loss) – measuring methods and dependence on washing procedure. In: Braun-Falco O, Korting HC (eds) Skin cleansing with synthetic detergents. Springer Verlag

Skin Hydration (Transepidermal Water Loss) – Measuring Methods and Dependence on Washing Procedure

H. Zienicke

Background

The stratum corneum (SC) has many functions, one of them being that of a barrier to protect the human body from external agents. Another aspect of the barrier function is the prevention of excessive loss of fluid, with the SC taking part in the body's fluid control mechanism. In this context, the hydration of the SC is of importance, and has been the subject of much research over the last decades.

Blank [3], the pioneer in this field, pointed out that the functional integrity of the skin is dependent on the moisture content of the SC. His studies showed that the skin will be soft and pliable for as long as the SC moisture content does not drop below 10 mg per 100 mg dry weight. If, because of low humidity, high ambient temperatures, or rapidly flowing air, the moisture content is reduced below that level, the skin will become brittle, chapped and rough – in other words, clinically dry. In a later paper, Blank [4] was able to show that the water binding and water holding capacity, and, hence, the structural integrity, of the SC are equally important for the flexibility and the appearance of the skin. These studies done by Blank paved the way for the development of techniques to measure skin hydration in vivo.

Over the last twenty years, the methods for the determination of SC water content have been complemented by techniques that allow the measurement of transepidermal water loss (TEWL) for the assessment of the integrity of the SC barrier function. The two parameters mentioned – SC water content, and TEWL – are important in studies of dry, rough, chapped skin, as has been shown in more recent investigations of the dry skin of atopic subjects. In patients with atopic eczema, the non-eczematized dry skin is due, not to a reduced water content in the upper horny layers [8, 10], but to a higher rate of flux through the skin because of a compromised water binding ability of the SC.

Determination of SC Water Content

The water content of the SC may be determined in vivo by measuring certain physical properties of the SC that are controlled by hydration and whose values, therefore, permit conclusions to be drawn as to the actual moisture content. The techniques that have been described involve the measurement of impedance [26, 37, 38, 41, 49, 50]; capacitance [41, 47]; resonance frequency [40, 41]; viscoelastic properties [25, 26]; and the use of infrared spectroscopy [10, 11] or photoacoustic spectroscopy [26].

However, since the hydration of the SC is non-uniform, and since each technique will measure water content at a different level of the SC, comparisons can be made only between results obtained by the same method. This dependence on the method used and the level examined was clearly shown by investigations of SC hydration in atopic subjects. Infrared spectroscopy [10] and impedance measurements as described by Lawler [8] of the dry skin of atopic subjects showed the upper SC to contain more water than the normal skin of healthy controls, while the use of the corneometer, measuring capacitance [47], showed a decreased water content as compared with normal controls.

The interest in measuring water loss from the human body goes back to the 17th century. At that time, people were weighed to determine how much water was lost every day [29]. Water is lost through the skin as a result of secretory perspiration (also known as sensible perspiration, or sweating); and as a result of insensible perspiration, i.e. the passive diffusion of water through the skin – a process also known as transepidermal water loss – and evaporation from the openings of the sweat glands, which, at temperatures below 31 °C, is, however, negligible. Thus, at temperatures below 31 °C, insensible perspiration can be taken to be the same as TEWL [22]. The level of TEWL is controlled by exogenous factors such as ambient humidity [2, 15, 16], environmental temperature [16], and skin temperature. Equally, there are controlling endogenous factors such as the thickness of the epidermis, as well as the surface texture and the water binding ability of the SC [8]. When the exogenous factors are kept constant, TEWL measurements will allow conclusions to be drawn as to the water binding ability of the SC [1, 7, 9, 23, 42].

This approach makes it possible to study the effects on the SC water binding ability of cosmetics, ointments, and irritants; and to assess the effects of treatment in such conditions as psoriasis [41] and atopic eczema [34].

Determination of TEWL

The techniques evolved for the in vivo measurement of TEWL are based upon two different principles.

In *non-ventilated techniques*, chemical or physical indicators are used to measure the increase in relative humidity in a capsule strapped to the skin. One chemical indicator is provided by filter paper impregnated with cobalt chloride, which is assessed with reflectance photometry. Semiconductors can be used to measure changes in resistance [41]. If hygroscopic salts such as calcium chloride [33] or magnesium perchlorate [16] are used, the weight change may be determined gravimetrically, or the change in relative humidity may be measured using an electrical hygrometer [28].

In the *ventilated technique*, the capsule is supplied with either a dry or a wet carrier gas at a constant flow rate, and the change in the water content of the gas is determined gravimetrically [2], electrohygrometrically [13], by infrared absorption [17], or by measuring the change in thermal conductivity [35].

Evaporimeter

The methods described above suffer from the disadvantage of requiring complex equipment and long measuring times; also, the skin is exposed to artificial ambient conditions. This is why Nilsson [24] developed an *evaporimeter*, which is superior in several respects to the methods previously used: The microclimate surrounding the skin surface is not disturbed, which means that, throughout the measurements, normal environmental conditions will prevail. Readings can be taken as little as 30 seconds after the application of the probe. The device is easy to handle and to operate. It consists of a meter and a probe, and is marketed by Servomed, Stockholm, Sweden. TEWL is computed automatically from the vapour pressure gradient above the skin, with a continuous digital display in g/m^2 h. The probe contains two pairs of sensors to measure relative humidity and temperature at two points. The sensors are arranged about 4 mm apart along the axis, and at 3 mm and 9 mm above the skin surface. They are protected by an open cylindrical PTFE capsule 15.5 mm high and 12.5 mm in diameter, which also serves to maintain a stable diffusion zone over the measuring site. The water vapour partial pressure is measured at each measuring point, and TEWL is derived from the pressure gradient. The technique is based upon the fact that the value of the vapour pressure gradient close to the skin surface, and, hence, to the moisture exchange, is approximately proportional to the difference between the vapour pressures measured at two discrete points along a line perpendicular to the surface and within the diffusion zone. At each point, the vapour pressure is computed from the product of the relative humidity and the saturated vapour pressure. Relative humidity is measured with the hygrometer, while the saturated vapour pressure, which is a function of temperature, is obtained from the temperature measured with the thermistor.

The accuracy of the evaporimeter as given by the manufacturer is 2 g/m^2 h. Blichmann et al. [6] were able to show that the accuracy of the device is three times the intra-individual coefficient of variation. In repeated studies in the same subject, they found a CV of 9.1%. Frödin et al. [9] were also able to show excellent reproducibility of the data obtained. Accuracy is affected by the contact pressure of the capsule on the skin surface, with a 10% increase in the evaporation rate for every 100 g of applied load. Consequently, the capsule should be very gently applied in order to keep the load below 40 g [24]. The measuring time is of lesser importance. The optimum recording time is stated to be 30 seconds after the application of the probe [6]. At high TEWL rates (above 75 g/m^2 h), the evaporimeter, as compared with a ventilated chamber, tends to underestimate the losses [31]. It is thought that this is due to an increase in the diffusion resistance of the probe, which significantly affects the diffusivity of the skin [48].

Unlike intra-individual variation, interindividual variation is high. Frödin et al. [9] studied TEWL on the backs of 10 women (mean age 30 years), and found an interindividual variation of 4–16 g/m² h. Blichmann et al. [6], in TEWL measurement on the forearm, also found a CV of 31–57%. Whereas, in general, no sex-related difference is reported [6, 44], Serup and Rasmussen [32] found significantly higher levels of TEWL on the dorsum of the hands of males as compared with females. Age also appears to influence the level of TEWL. Serup and Rasmussen [32] found decreases in evaporation with increasing age. Even if the environmental conditions in terms of humidity and ambient temperature are kept approximately constant, other exogenous factors such as the use of emollients [32], or washing habits, may influence the level of water loss, as will be shown below, in the section on our studies. This would explain why measurements obtained using identical methods and performed at the same sites may lead to different results [6, 39, 46]. Regional differences in the TEWL values obtained by such authors as Ude [44] (who attributed the differences to different skin temperatures), or by Dupuis et al. [7] (who found these differences to persist even after correcting to a common skin temperature of 30 °C) have been considered as being due to regional differences in skin thickness [32] and SC thickness [18], or to differences in corneocyte size and horny layer patterns at different sites [7]. Sebum on the skin surface is thought to have no influence on TEWL [19].

Effect of Soaps and Synthetic Detergents on Skin Hydration

Background

While the earliest known formula for a soap-like substance goes back to the third millenium B.C., skin care as we know it was not introduced until around 1700 A.D. Soap came to be increasingly used in the first third of the 19th century, and further progress in personal hygiene was made when synthetic detergents were developed [30].

The skin has to be cleansed from time to time to remove foreign substances such as dust and grime, and to get rid of substances produced or shed by the skin itself, such as sweat, oil, and desquamating cells. For this purpose, soap and synthetic detergents are used. Both types of agents contain surfactants that provide the detersive action [36]. Apart from their intended cleansing effect, these agents also have a number of unwanted effects, which are related to the concentration of the washing solution and to the time of exposure [43]. Blank and Shappirio [5] were engaged in in-vitro studies of the effects of soap and synthetic detergents as early as 1955. They were able to show that after cornified epithelium had been treated with soap or synthetic detergents, the water binding ability of the SC was reduced, because of the removal, by the washing process, of water soluble substances – especially amino acids – from the horny layer.

Vermeer et al. [45] determined the amounts of dissolved amino acids after washing as a function of the pH of the buffer solution used, and found that at a high pH more amino acids were extracted from the horny layer than was the case at lower pH levels. The *short-term and long-term effects on SC hydration of an arm bath* in either a soap or a synthetic detergent solution have been studied in vivo using DC conductance measurements [50], infrared spectroscopy [11, 12], the resonance frequency technique [40], and measurements of capacitance [12]. Infrared spectroscopy showed a hydration effect immediately after bathing of the arm in either the soap or the synthetic detergent solution; at ten minutes, moisture values lower than those before washing were seen only with soap. DC conductance measurements after bathing in synthetic detergent solution also showed initial hydration followed 30 minutes later by a drop in water content to below pre-bathing values [50]. Tronnier [43], using the resonance frequency technique with reference to water, showed that after bathing in alkaline (pH 9 and pH 11) buffer solutions, there was initially much hydration, followed by slight drying later on; after bathing in buffer solutions adjusted to an acid or a neutral pH (pH 2, 4, or 7), he observed marked drying not preceded by hydration. Gloor et al. [12] studied the long-term SC hydration effects, after four days, of three daily immersions in soap or synthetic detergent solutions. Using infrared spectroscopy and capacitance measurements, these authors were able to show that dehydration is more prolonged after bathing in a soap solution than in a synthetic detergent one. Whereas two hours after the last detergent bath, pre-bathing levels had been restored after initial significant dehydration, no rehydration could be observed in those who had been bathing in a soap solution.

Most of the studies performed in the past have looked at the effect of a single washing; also, in-vivo studies to date have been concerned with the water content of, rather than with water loss through, the SC. We therefore decided that our study [21] should investigate the *effects on TEWL of repeated washing with synthetic detergents of different pHs*. Since washing with these agents may be expected to result not only in a change in the water binding ability of the SC, but also in pH changes [20] and greater skin roughness [43], it was decided to study the three parameters in parallel. In order to enable intra-individual comparisons to be made, the cross-over design [20] previously used by our team was adopted.

Material and methods are described by D. Vieluf elsewhere in this monograph, in the chapter on skin roughness.

Our Results

This paper contains the preliminary results of the study described above [21], with the main emphasis on the TEWL aspects of the investigation.

At the forehead site (Fig. 1), repeated intensive washing with a pH 5.5 or a pH 8.5 synthetic detergent cleanser leads to a rapid increase in TEWL. After some two to three weeks, a steady state is reached, with the TEWL levelling off. Following the cross-over to the other cleanser, there is an initial phase during

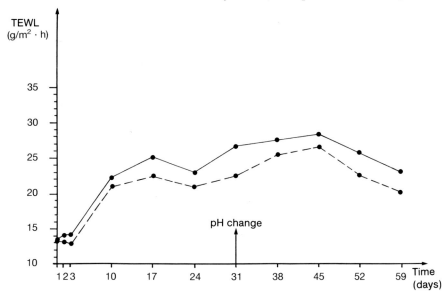

Fig. 1. Forehead TEWL in the pH 5.5 (———) and pH 8.5 (– – – –) groups

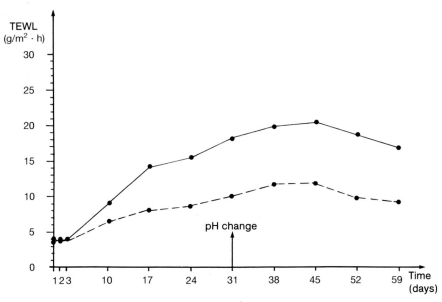

Fig. 2. Forearm TEWL in the pH 5.5 (———) and pH 8.5 (– – – –) groups

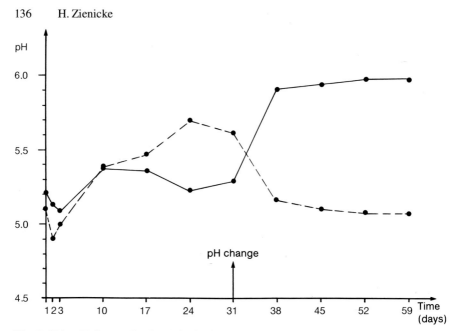

Fig. 3. Skin pH change (forehead) in the pH 5.5 (———) and pH 8.5 (– – – –) groups

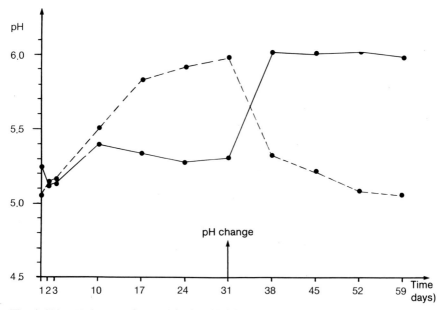

Fig. 4. Skin pH changes (forearm) in the pH 5.5 (———) and pH 8.5 (– – – –) groups

which, once again, the water loss is increased; again, this is followed by a levelling off of TEWL after another two to three weeks. A comparison between the two groups shows the two graphs to be more or less parallel at the forehead site, without any significant difference between the groups. At the forearm site, the pattern is different, as will be seen from the group comparison shown in Figure 2. It would appear that after intensive washing with the pH 5.5 cleanser, there is a greater increase in TEWL on the forearm than can be seen following the use of the pH 8.5 cleanser; however, this does not necessarily mean that the effect seen is significantly dependent on the pH of the skin cleansing preparation used. By the time of cross-over, 28 days after the subjects started using the cleanser, there is no clear-cut evidence of levelling off. Following cross-over, the pattern in both groups is like the one seen at the forehead site, with forearm TEWL values going on rising, and an eventual return to lower levels. Longer-term studies will have to be done in order to find out whether, given sufficient time, the TEWL returns to pre-trial values, or whether it steadies out at a level above the baseline water loss. A comparison of the trial phase skin pH patterns at the forehead site (Fig. 3) and at the forearm site (Fig. 4) with the patterns of TEWL (Figs. 1 and 2) does not show a close correlation between TEWL and skin pH.

Our studies confirm the in-vitro results of Blank and Shappirio [5], who found that washing with synthetic detergents may result in an increase in TEWL.

Our study also suggests a difference between the forehead and the forearm sites, with the latter possibly producing a greater increase in TEWL in response to intensive washing with an acidic detergent than after the use of a more alkaline agent. Further studies should be designed to establish whether this difference really does exist, and whether the phenomenon may be at least partially attributable to the higher lipid content of the forehead skin.

References

1. Abe T (1978) Studies on skin surface barrier functions. Transepidermal water loss and skin surface lipids during childhood. Chem Pharm Bull 26: 1659–1665
2. Bettley FR, Grice KA (1967) The influence of ambient humidity on transepidermal water loss. Brit J Dermatol 79: 575–581
3. Blank IH (1952) Factors with influence the water content of the stratum corneum. J Invest Dermatol 18: 433–440
4. Blank IH (1953) Further observations on factors which influence the water content of the stratum corneum. J Invest Dermatol 21: 259–271
5. Blank IH, Shappiro EB (1955) The water content of the stratum corneum. J Invest Dermatol 25: 391–401
6. Blichmann CW, Serup J (1987) Reproducibility and variability of transepidermal water loss measurement. Studies on the ServoMed Evaporimeter. Acta Derm Venereol (Stockh) 67: 206–210
7. Dupuis D, Rougier A, Lotte C, Wilson DR, Maibach HJ (1986) In vivo relationship between percutaneous absorption and transepidermal water loss according to anatomic site in man. J Soc Cosmet Chem 37: 351–357
8. Finlay AY, Nicholls S, King CS, Marks R (1980) The "dry" non-eczematous skin associated with atopic eczema. Brit J Dermatol 102: 249–256

9. Frödin T, Skogh M (1984) Measurement of transepidermal water loss using an evaporimeter to follow the restitution of the barrier layer of human epidermis after stripping the stratum corneum. Acta Derm Venereol (Stockh) 64: 537–540
10. Gloor M, Heymann B, Stuhlert T (1981) Infrared spectroscopic determination of the water content of the horny layer in healthy subjects and in patients suffering from atopic dermatitis. Arch Dermatol Res 271: 429–436
11. Gloor M, Hirsch G, Willebrandt U (1981) On the use of infrared spectroscopy for the in vivo measurement of the water content of the horny layer after application of dermatologic ointments. Arch Dermatol Res 271: 305–313
12. Gloor M, Gehse M, Wölfle N (1985) Beeinflussung der Hornschichtfeuchtigkeit durch waschaktive Substanzen. Ärztl Kosmetol 15: 293–302
13. Grice K, Bettley RF (1967) The effect of skin temperature and vascular change on the rate of transepidermal water loss. Brit J Dermatol 79: 582–588
14. Grice K, Sattar H, Sharatt M, Baker H (1971) Skin temperature and transepidermal water loss. J Invest Dermatol 57: 108–110
15. Grice K, Sattar H, Baker H (1972) The effect of ambient humidity on transepidermal water loss. J Invest Dermatol 58: 343–346
16. Hattingh J (1972) The influence of skin temperature, environmental temperature and relative humidity on transepidermal water loss. Acta Derm Venereol (Stockh) 52: 438–440
17. Johnson C, Shuster S (1969) The measurement of transepidermal water loss. Brit J Dermatol 81, Suppl 4: 40–46
18. Klaschka F (1974) Hautoberflächendiagnostik und ihre klinische Relevanz. Zeitschr Hautkr 49: 811–817
19. Kligman AM (1983) The use of sebum. Brit J Dermatol 75: 307–319
20. Korting HC, Kober M, Mueller M, Braun-Falco O (1987) Influence of repeated washings with soap and synthetic detergents on pH and resident flora of the skin of forehead and forearm. Results of a cross-over trial in healthy probitioners. Acta Derm Venereol (Stockh) 67: 41–47
21. Korting HC, Megele M, Mehringer L, Vieluf D, Zienicke H, Hamm G (in preparation) Influence of repeated washings with an acide and an alcaline synthetic detergent of identical chemical composition on pH, roughness and transepidermal water loss of forehead and forearm. Acta Derm Venereol (Stockh)
22. Morsches B (1980) Anorganische Chemie der Haut. In: Dermatologie in Praxis und Klinik, Korting GW (ed) Vol 1 pp 3.1–3.10, Thieme Verlag, Stuttgart New York
23. Neste van D, Masmoudi M, Leroy B, Mahmoud G, Lachapelle JM (1986) Regression patterns of transepidermal water loss and of cutaneous blood flow values in sodium lauryl sulfate induced irritation: a human model of rough dermatitic skin. Bioeng Skin 2: 103–118
24. Nilsson GE (1977) Measurement of water exchange through skin. Med & Biol Eng & Comput 15: 209–218
25. Potts RO, Buras EM, Chrisman DA (1984) Changes with age in the moisture content of human skin. J Invest Dermatol 82: 97–100
26. Potts RO (1986) Stratum corneum hydration: experimental techniques and interpretations of results. J Soc Cosmet Chem 37: 9–33
27. Rajyka G (1974) Transepidermal water loss on the hands in atopic dermatitis. Arch Dermatol Forsch 251: 111–115
28. Rosenberg EW, Blank H, Resnik S (1962) Sweating and water loss trough the skin. Amer Med Ass 179: 809–811
29. Sanctorius (1720) Medicina statica, 2nd Edn, quoted in 23
30. Schneider W, Tronnier H, Wagner H (1962) Reinigung und Pflege der Haut im Beruf unter besonderer Berücksichtigung der experimentellen und praktischen Prüfverfahren. In: Dermatologie und Venerologie, Gottron A, Schönfeld W (eds) Vol 1, Part 2, pp 1043–1100, Thieme Verlag, Stuttgart
31. Scott RC, Oliver GJA, Dugard PH, Singh HJ (1982) A comparison of techniques for the measurement of transepidermal water loss. Arch Dermatol Res 274: 57–64

32. Serup J, Rasmussen I (1985) Dry hands in scleroderma. Acta Derm Venerol (Stockh) 65: 419–423
33. Shahidullah M, Raffle EJ, Frain-Bell W (1967) Insensible water loss in dermatitis. Brit J Dermatol 79: 589–597
34. Shahidullah M, Raffle EJ, Rimmer AR, Frain-Bell W (1969) Transepidermal water loss in patients with dermatitis. Brit J Dermatol 81: 722–730
35. Spruit D (1967) Measurement of the water vapour loss from human skin by a thermal conductivity cell. J Appl Physiol 23: 994–997
36. Stüttgen G (1965) Der Wassergehalt der Haut. In: Die normale und pathologische Physiologie der Haut, pp 234–250, Fischer, Stuttgart
37. Tagami H, Ohi, M, Iwatsuki K, Kanamaru Y, Yamada M, Ichijo B (1980) Evaluation of the skin surface hydration in vivo by electrical measurement. J Invest Dermatol 75: 500–507
38. Tagami H, Ohi M, Iwatsuki K, Yamada M (1983) Electrical measurement of the hydration state of the skin surface in vivo. In: Stratum corneum, Marks R, Plewig G (Eds), pp 252–256, Springer, Berlin Heidelberg
39. Triebskorn A, Gloor M, Greiner F (1983) Comparative investigations on the water content of the stratum corneum using different methods of measurement. Dermatologica 167: 64–69
40. Tronnier H, Kuhn-Bussius H (1963) Kritische Übersicht zur Frage der Messung der Resonanzfrequenz der Haut unter Berücksichtigung der Auswertung und der Streubreite der Methodik. Arch Klin Exp Dermatol 217: 563–576
41. Tronnier H (1980) Differenzierte Feuchtigkeitsmessungen an der menschlichen Haut. Ärztl Kosmetol 10: 291–308
42. Tronnier H (1981) Vergleichende Messungen der Hornschichthydratation. Fette Seifen Anstrichm 83: 442–449
43. Tronnier H (1985) Seifen und Syndets in der Hautpflege und -therapie. Ärztl Kosmetol 15: 19–30
44. Ude P (1978) Physikalische Hautmeßwerte und ihre topographischen Unterschiede. Ärztl Kosmetol 8: 221–227
45. Vermeer DJH, Jong de JC, Donk LA (1966) Skin damage by washing. Dermatologica 132: 305–319
46. Werner Y, Lindberg M (1985) Transepidermal water loss in dry and clinically normal skin in patients with atopic dermatitis. Acta Derm Venereol (Stockh) 65: 102–105
47. Werner Y (1986) The water content of the stratum corneum in patients with atopic dermatitis. Acta Derm Venereol (Stockh) 66: 281–284
48. Wheldon AE, Monteith JL (1980) Performance of a skin evaporimeter. Med & Biol Eng & Comput 18: 201–205
49. Wienert V, Hegner G, Sick H (1981) Ein Verfahren zur Bestimmung des relativen Wassergehaltes des Stratum corneum der menschlichen Haut. Arch Dermatol Res 270: 67–75
50. Wienert V, Sick H (1982) Ein neues Meßgerät zur routinemäßigen Bestimmung der Hautfeuchtigkeit. Ärztl Kosmetol 12: 416–422

Beneficial Effects of Synthetic Detergent Cleansers in Human Trials Under Simulated Use Conditions

Cleansing Action of Synthetic Detergents – Methodology of Determination

K. Schrader

Background

In the assessment of cleansing products, soil removal is of prime importance. The detersive action must be exerted in such a way as to ensure that, during washing, only the superficial water-lipid mantle is removed. In other words, there should be only temporary replacement of the soil/water-lipid mantle/skin interface by the cleanser/skin interface. At the same time, any water or lipids that have been removed should be restored, and the water holding capacity of the stratum corneum, as well as the buffer envelope, should be regenerated.

In general, no one surfactant or mixture of surfactants would be able to meet these requirements.

Inevitably, the physiological milieu will be disturbed, and will have to be restored by appropriate skin care after cleansing [1].

Methods

A number of methods for testing the defatting and detersive actions of cleansers have been described.

One in-vitro method frequently employed in the assessment of the degreasing action of surfactants uses woollen yarn [2]. It should, however, be remembered that this method will give gravimetric information on the lipophilic constituents of the soil only.

Würbach has described a method of extracting and determining skin lipids before and after washing, using a special device known as a washing bell, which is applied to the back of the subject [3]. Once again, it is the skin lipids rather than the whole "soil spectrum" that is detected.

Tronnier [4] became interested early on in testing the detersive power of surfactants in the human skin. He produced the model soil described below, which we have found to be reasonably representative of all the types of soil encountered. The soil formula is based upon a W/O emulsion containing a lipid and a water soluble dye, as well as a pigment to represent mineral soil (Table 1).

The washing device contains a rotating plastic agitator. The chief criticism of the experimental apparatus is the fact that rotation causes different circumferen-

Table 1. Formula of model soil ointment, W/O emulsion

Ingredient	%	Supplier
Sicomet Red F (C.I. 12150) (lipid soluble)	4.0	BASF, Ludwigshafen
Sicovit Cochineal Red 70 E 124		BASF, Ludwigshafen
(C.I. 16255) (water soluble)	4.0	BASF, Ludwigshafen
Sicomet Red P (C.I. 12490) (Pigment)	4.0	Th. Goldschmidt, Essen
Protegin	17.0	Th. Goldschmidt, Essen
Tegin 0 spezial	2.5	Rova, Duisburg
Stellux A.I.	5.5	H. E. Wagner, Bremen
Liquid light paraffin	6.5	H. E. Wagner, Bremen
White soft paraffin	10.0	
Water, demineralized	46.5	
	100.0	

tial velocities of the liquor in the test area. This means that the skin is exposed to different mechanical washing intensities, which may be a source of errors.

Since the methods described above, as well as others known to us, are frequently rather unrealistic, we decided to design our own skin washing simulator (Fig. 1).

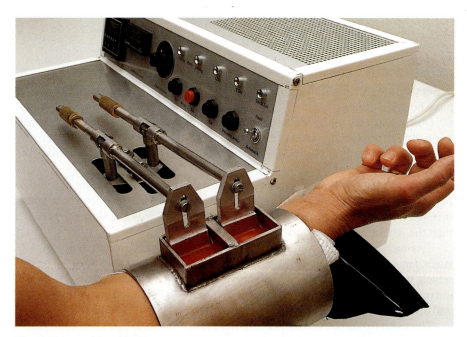

Fig. 1. Skin washing simulator

Principle of the Skin Washing Simulator

The machine simulates the washing process by the to-and-fro movement of scrubbing arms with felt blades.

Equipment Description

Two parallel mounted, eccentrically driven scrubbing arms with needle felt blades are moved to and fro over the skin of the forearm, maintaining a preset contact pressure and working at a defined speed.

An inflatable cuff within the device ensures that the forearm is pressed against the two parallel chambers that are filled with the detergent solutions. The skin thus provides a natural seal. The chambers are filled with defined volumes of the detergent solutions to be tested, and the scrubbing units are mounted on their shafts. The device is now ready for use.

Performance of the Test

a) A rubber stamp is applied to the volar side of the forearm to mark the test areas (field size: 4.0 cm by 4.0 cm) (Fig. 2).

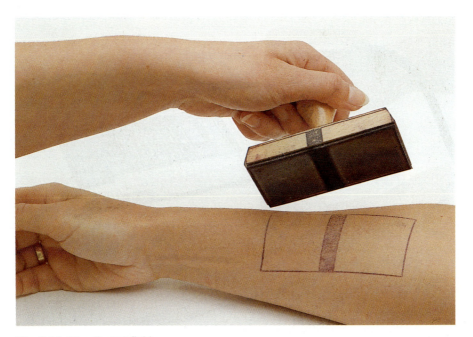

Fig. 2. Marking the test fields

b) The colour of the skin is determined using a colorimeter (CR 200 Chromameter, Minolta, Hamburg) (3 measurements per test field; mean = Value 1) (Fig. 3).
c) Model soil (50 mg) is applied with a spatula (Fig. 4).
d) The soil is allowed to dry for 10 minutes, at room temperature.
e) The degree of skin soiling is measured (3 measurements per test field; mean Value = 2).
f) The cuff in the washing device is inflated to press the forearm against the two parallel mounted detergent receptacles (washing chambers), with the skin forming a natural seal.
g) Each 24 mL chamber is filled with 5 mL of the detergent solutions to be tested (temperature of test solutions: 23 °C) (Fig. 5).
h) The scrubbing arms with felt blades are inserted into the washing chambers. The contact load of the arms on the skin of the forearm is 16 g, and the contact angle is 90°.
i) The scrubbing arms are moved to and fro at constant speed to simulate the frictional process involved in washing of the skin (48 strokes/min); the total washing time is 60 seconds (Fig. 6).
k) The test products are removed from the chambers.
l) The washed areas are allowed to dry for 10 minutes.
m) The washed area is measured (3 measurements per test field; mean Value = 3) (Fig. 7).

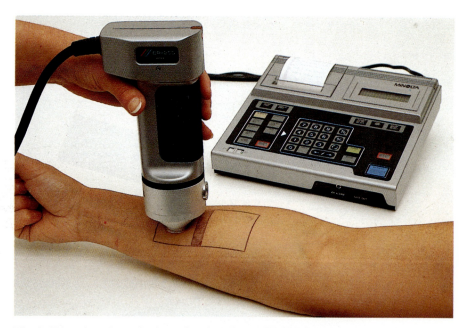

Fig. 3. Skin colour determination using the Minolta CR 200 chromameter

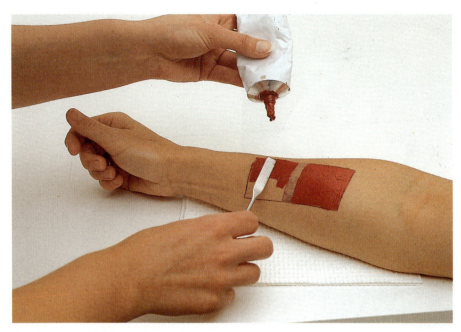

Fig. 4. Application of model soil

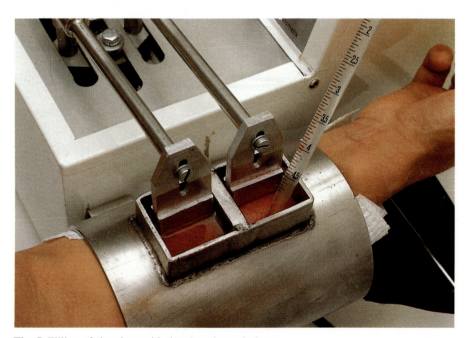

Fig. 5. Filling of chambers with the cleansing solutions

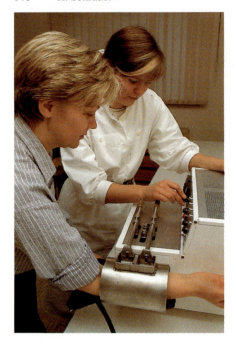

Fig. 6. Simulated washing

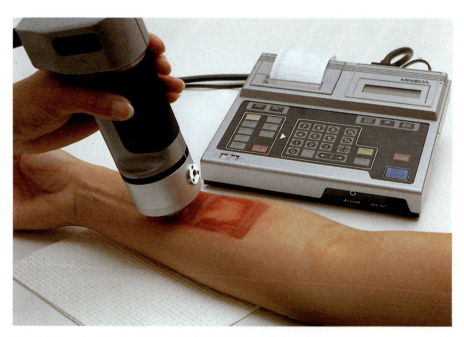

Fig. 7. Measuring the washed area with the Minolta CR 200 chromameter

n) The three values are used to calculate the amount of soil removed by the washing process:

$$\frac{\text{Value 3 minus Value 2}}{\text{Value 1 minus Value 2}} \cdot 100 = \text{Detergency [\%]}$$

The following criteria have been standardized (cf. Table 2):

Table 2. Standardized criteria

– Test field size	4.0 cm by 4.0 cm
– Model soil composition	see Formula (Table 1)
– Amount applied	50 mg
– Model soil drying time	10 min at room temperature
– Test solution volume	5 mL
– Test solution temperature	23 °C
– Test chamber volume	24 mL
– Type of felt	needle felt
– Contact load	16 g
– Contact angle	90°
– Speed	48 strokes/min
– Washing time	60 sec

Experiments

Washing Trials

Ten healthy volunteers (6 females, 4 males, aged 14 to 52) were enrolled. Since the results obtained are well reproducible, 10 subjects should, as a rule, be enough. The substances tested were 3 commercially available shower bath preparations, whose characteristics are shown in Table 3.

Table 3. Product analysis

Code	pH 10 % sol.	Surfactant content [%]	NaCl content [%]
6	6.3	22.0	1.85
31	7.2	22.0	2.13
37	6.3	25.0	1.78
Texapon K 12	6–9 (1% sol.)	90.5 min.	2 max.

These shower bath preparations were tested against sodium lauryl sulphate 2% dissolved in water of 8° German hardness, and against water of 8° German hardness.

Additional Tests

In order to assess some of the "side effects," skin roughness and ocular irritancy were included as additional parameters.

It was assumed that surfactants have different affinities for skin and mucous membranes, which frequently result in adverse effects. In order to evaluate such events, we used an in-vitro alternative (non-animal) method for the assessment of acute irritation.

The determination of human skin roughness in 20 subjects using the methylene blue technique has been modified by us [5]. The test was done with 2% solutions of the products.

In-vitro Ocular Irritancy Test

Ocular irritancy was assessed by studying the haemolysis and denaturation of bovine blood [6] (Fig. 8).

This test measures the destruction of blood cells and the release of oxyhaemoglobin as a measure of the typical irritant effects of surfactants on intact cell structures. The two parameters are associated in an index, which provides a ready means of assessing and classifying detergents, and which correlates well with in-vivo methods such as the Draize test. In the haemolysis test, photometry

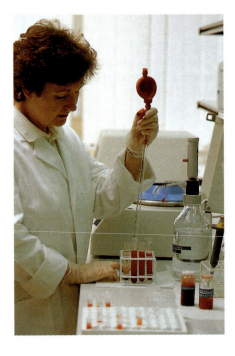

Fig. 8. In-vitro irritancy test

is used to determine the detergent concentration (in μl/mL of surfactant) that will lyse 50% of the bovine red blood cells in isotonic buffer.

The denaturation of a 1% detergent solution of bovine haemoglobin is also assessed photometrically.

The two parameters H (haemolysis) and D (denaturation) are used to calculate the final MIOI (**M**ean **I**ndex of **O**cular **I**rritation), which correlates very well with the Draize test (Table 4).

Table 4. Classification of irritancy

MIOI	Level
<5	non-irritant
5–15	mildly irritant
15–30	irritant
>30	very irritant

Methylene Blue Method

The stratum corneum may be expected to adsorb greater or lesser quantities of the dye methylene blue, depending on surface roughness (Fig. 9).

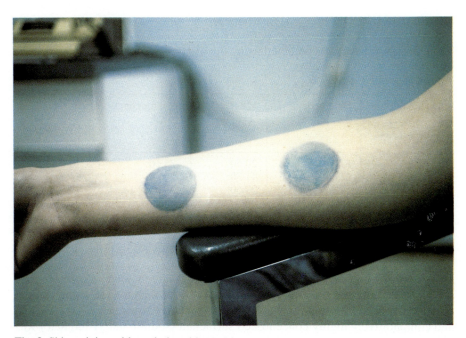

Fig. 9. Skin staining with methylene blue

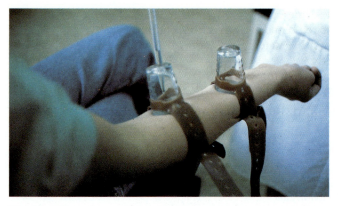

Fig. 10. Filling of cups with wash solutions

After the dye has been extracted from the skin with detergent, the amount of dye is measured spectrophotometrically (Fig. 10).

The results are used to calculate roughness in per cent, e.g. of the initial value. The values obtained are normalized, with a 2% sodium lauryl sulphate solution taken to produce 100% roughness. A confidence range of 95% is given as the measure of dispersion.

Results and Discussion

Table 5 shows the results obtained using the method described above.

Table 5. Results

Product 2%	Detergency	MIOI	Skin roughness	
			Mean (n = 20)	Confidence range
6	57.33	20.60	35.50	14.7
31	61.77	41.30	74.70	11.8
37	57.93	29.60	55.50	13.7
Water	43.68	–	–	–
Texapon K 12 (2% in water)	75.24	–	100.0	–

All the three products showed pronounced detergency. As expected, they produced a result that was highly significantly better than that of water, even at detergent concentrations as low as 0.3 to 0.4% active substance (AS). A harsh and comparatively highly concentrated surfactant (sodium lauryl sulphate) was able to increase detergency by only ca. 15%.

We were struck by the absence of any significant difference between the various shower bath preparations. A paired t-test showed p >0.1 [7]. All the products are in the 60% detergency range.

While detergency was similar, there was a difference in the MIOI by almost 2 irritancy levels between Products 6 and 31. Product 6 was found to be close to the "mildly irritant" level (MIOI <15), whereas Product 31 proved to be a "very irritant" shower bath formulation. Since, as a rule, the relative error of MIOI values is less than 10%, the difference found is significant.

The three products also differed significantly in their skin roughness values (p <0.05).

In summary, it is possible to formulate detergents to make them non-irritating to the skin and mucous membranes without any major loss of cleansing action. A mild product can be made to give about the same cleaning performance as a much more irritant product.

Conclusions

The skin washing simulator works under well standardized and largely realistic conditions to yield data that lend themselves to a ready analysis of the skin detergency of surfactant products. Products with a good cleansing performance can subsequently be classified in terms of their irritancy.

The skin washing simulator is also very adaptable. Various characteristics of the set-up can be modified for the study of other aspects, such as the removal of make-up or of occupational hand soiling, with special cleansers and specially formulated model soils.

References

1. Schrader K (1984) Vergleichende Prüfungen über die Hautreinigung in Bezug auf die Verträglichkeit von Tensiden. Parfümerie und Kosmetik 65: 671–674, 676
2. Modde H, Schuster G, Tronnier H (1965) Experimentelle Untersuchungen zum Problem der Hautverträglichkeit anionaktiver Tenside in der Arbeitsmedizin. Tenside 2: 368–373
3. Würbach G (1981) Entfettung der Hautoberfläche durch Tenside in Abhängigkeit von Konzentration und Konstitution. Cosmetics Symposium, Halle (GDR)
4. Tronnier H (1965) Zur Standardisierung von Waschversuchen an der menschlichen Haut. Fette, Seifen, Anstrichmittel 67: 7
5. Padberg N (1969) Modifizierte Methylenblau-Methode zur Prüfung des Rauhigkeitsgrades der Hornschicht. J Soc Cosm Chem 20: 719–728
6. Pape JW, Hoppe U (1988) 2nd World Tenside Congress 1988, Vol 4, pp 414–428
7. Sachs L (1984) Angewandte Statistik, Springer-Verlag, 6th ed, pp 242–244

Clinical Assessment of Synthetic Detergent Cleansers in Subjects with Problem Skin

F. Klaschka

Introduction

Synthetic detergent cleansers have been formulated to clean as well as, or better than, conventional soap, while being optimally tolerated by those whose hands and fingers are exposed to occupational irritants, and by those who suffer from "problem" skin that is easily irritated or tends to be affected by eczema. Soap-free cleanser concentrates provide an alternative for those who cannot tolerate soap, and are widely used for the cleansing and care of normal and of diseased skin. In fact, synthetic cleansers used in conjunction with topical dermatological agents may be regarded as a disease modifying management principle [1, 2, 4] for patients with problem skin. In this context, "problem skin" means skin that tends to be abnormally sensitive or irritable, such as the skin of atopics, especially those suffering from neurodermatitis, or skin with pre- or post-eczematous lesions (both exogenous or endogenous eczema) that require care and/or treatment.

Clinical Assessment

By their very nature, acidic synthetic cleansers help to restore the protective "acid mantle" of the skin. Extensive and sophisticated studies have been performed, in vivo or in models [5], to establish whether synthetic cleansers can do better than conventional (alkaline) soap when it comes to cleaning "normal" or "problem" skins.

In addition to the quantification of the *cleansing power* in the form of a mean "detergency" value of the raw material surfactants or the finished detergent formulation, great efforts have been made to use colorimetric or profilometric methods to establish the *skin compatibility*, i.e. the non-irritancy, of substances and products. Detergents can damage the skin by diminishing the water holding capacity of the stratum corneum, which means that the initial swelling of the horny layer will be followed by drying, with increased loosening and detachment of peripheral corneocytes. This process manifests itself by scaling and flaking, a loss of skin flexibility, and an increased permeability of the stratum corneum for solvents and chemical agents that may act as irritants. Anionic detergents notoriously cause an unpleasant "detergent feel," which is due to the salt-like binding of the detergent to the skin, leading to swelling of the horny layer. While still damp, the stratum corneum will feel "tacky"; two hours later, once it has become fully dry and the swelling has subsided, the skin will, as a rule, feel more or less "rough" – witness the rough hands of housewives, who have to steep their hands in detergent solutions for many of their chores. Fatty agents offer some protection against this roughness.

Test Methods

Chief among the methods for the clinical assessment of the efficacy and the irritancy potential of synthetic cleansers are realistic tests (use tests) performed in large groups of subjects. In one such test, a soap-free, moisturizing synthetic cleanser concentrate, pH-5-Eucerin Waschlotio® (Beiersdorf, Hamburg, FRG), was used in 60 patients, most of whom were suffering from eczema at the healing stage. These patients were enrolled into a wash test that involved the twice daily use, for two weeks, of the lotion, in order to assess the suitability of the preparation in the aftercare of eczematous conditions of different origin [4] and in the postinflammatory stage of other skin disorders. The unselected patient group consisted of 45 females and 15 males, aged between 18 and 79. Of the 60 volunteers, 43 had allergic or irritant contact dermatitis; 12 had neurodermatitis; and 4 had other inflammatory skin disorders (3 cases of psoriasis; 1 case of sensitive and irritated senile skin) (Table 1).

The study was performed in order to obtain a rational assessment of the side-effect profile of the cleanser, in normal and in diseased skin, under conditions of twice-daily use for two weeks, during which time those of the patients who had been prescribed dermatological medication or preparations were also

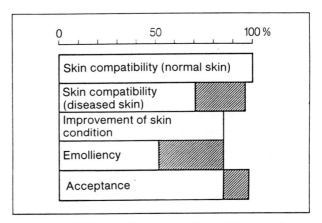

Fig. 1. Overall assessment of the beneficial effects or pH 5-Eucerin-Waschlotio. *Open bars* = Total of Very Good and Good ratings. *Hatched areas* = Fair ratings [4]

Table 1. Patient population. Skin disorders and symptoms

Skin disorders	Patients (n)
Exogenous eczema	43
Endogenous eczema	12
Other skin disorders	4
Senile skin	1
Symptoms	Reported
Scaling	33
(Residual) redness	29
Dry skin	26
Cracking	15
Brittleness	8
Lichenification	5
Itching	4
Erosion	1
Roughness	1
Stinging	1

using their ointments, creams, lotions, or gels. In this patient population with constitutionally sensitive and/or eczematous dry, scaling, fissured skins, particular attention was paid to any changes observed in the condition of the skin during the use of pH-5-Eucerin®-Waschlotio, to detect both improvements and unwanted effects; also, patients were asked to report on how they were using the cleanser in conjunction with any other topical agents they had been prescribed.

Results

For the study of skin compatibility, the patients were classified according to disease severity. The symptom list in Table 1 was used in the assessment of irritancy, in involved and non-involved skin areas. The statistical analysis of the irritancy results was done using the Student t-test [6] and the (one-sided) Wilcoxon-Mann-Whitney U-test [6], to establish the significance of any differences observed. The results have been summarized in Table 2. In mild or moderate skin disease, the cleanser was tolerated well or very well in 66.6% of the cases. Even in severe skin disease, tolerability was good to fair. One patient suffering from dyshidrotic eczema reported transient stinging when using the cleansing lotion; this result was classified as "poor." Overall, the product was less well tolerated by patients suffering from dyshidrotic eczema with red, scaling, cracked skin; however, the difference was not significant.

A comparison between the side effects in normal skin areas and those in areas affected by different severities of skin disease shows a highly significant difference between normal skin and severely affected areas. There is a marked dependence of the irritancy of the cleanser on the severity of the skin disorders.

Table 2. Assessment of skin compatibility of the cleansing lotion

A. Compatibility with diseased skin as a function of disease severity: Good to fair tolerability in 6/7 cases; even in severely affected areas

Ratings[a]	Severity — Diseased skin		
	mild	moderate	severe
Very good	8 (13.3%)	5 (8.3%)	–
Good	4 (6.7%)	23 (38.3%)	2 (3.3%)
Fair	–	13 (21.7%)	4 (6.7%)
Poor	–	–	1 (1.7%)

B. Compatibility with normal skin areas of patients suffering from different severities of skin disease[b]

Rating	Severity		
	mild	moderate	severe
Very good	9 (15%)	14 (23%)	2 (3.3%)
Good	3 (5%)	27 (45%)	5 (8%)

C. Adverse effects as a function of disease severity

Symptoms	Severity		
	mild	moderate	severe
Stinging	–	2 (3.3%)	3 (5.0%)
Smarting	–	–	1 (1.7%)

[a] Highly significant difference
[b] No significant dependence

There was no correlation between the response of the non-involved areas and the severity of disease in the involved areas.

Irritant effects in diseased skin manifested themselves by stinging when the cleanser was first used; this irritancy was markedly dependent on the severity of skin disease. While patients reported that the cleanser was tolerated very well in 42%, and well in 58% of the cases in normal skin areas, Very good and Good ratings together accounted for 70% of the assessments in the diseased areas. If the category of Fair ratings is included, the total percentage of favourable ratings is 95%.

The *effect on skin lesions* was reported as "Improved" in 51 cases; "No Change" in 9 cases; while "Worse" was not reported in any of the cases. Of the "No Change" cases, one was being treated concurrently with a steroid cream, and the other one with uncoloured Castellani's paint. These two cases were excluded from the analysis. 29 out of 33 contact dermatitis patients were improved. Of the 5 cases of dyshidrotic eczema, only two were improved, the other 3 were unchanged.

Of the 60 patients in the study, 51 reported an *emollient effect*, which was rated "Very Good" or "Good" in 31 cases (51%), and was perceived equally in endogenous and in exogenous eczema. Apart from the cleansing lotion, 2 patients were using dermatological medication, and 33 patients (55%) some sort of skin care agent. 25 patients (52%) were using neither medication nor skin care preparations. It was interesting to note that 6 of the 7 "No Change" cases had been using skin care preparations in addition to the cleanser, while 24 of the 51 who were "Improved" had not used any other skin care agents.

Assessment and Discussion

This example of a use study shows how a soap-free cleanser can be assessed for (gentle) cleansing and, above all, for its compatibility with problem skin, i.e. chiefly constitutionally sensitive and dry skin, as well as eczema at the healing stage. After pH-5-Eucerin®-Waschlotio had been used for two weeks, on average twice a day, it was found that out of 60 patients (mainly subjects recovering from eczema), 59 (98%) had found the cleanser pleasant to use, and of these, 51 (85%) had tolerated the product well or very well, on non-involved as well as on involved skin areas. The emollient effect of the preparation on the treated areas, and the efficacy of the cleanser in helping to clear up the eczema were stressed by 51 of the 60 patients (mainly subjects suffering from contact dermatitis or neurodermatitis). Even post-eczematous skin was not irritated or aggravated, which would confirm earlier reports that, unlike soap, soap-less cleanser concentrates only rarely produce irritation in eczema patients [1, 2, 3]. Since the synthetic cleansers do no possess the Ca^{++} and Mg^{++} precipitating properties of soap, any irritation that may initially occur will be comparatively mild. If the lotion is applied directly to cracks or erosions, there may be some transient stinging or smarting; however, there appears to be no itching and/or inflammation [2, 4]. The cleansing lotion was well received by the overwhelming majority (85%) of the patients. This acceptance, which is vital for good patient compliance, underlines the great efficacy and good skin compatibility of this synthetic cleanser. The cleansing lotion described here is typical of synthetic cleansers in general, as agents that cleanse mildly but thoroughly, thus meeting the dermatologists's requirements for a product that will afford skin care and protection.

References

1. Braun-Falco O, Heilgemeir P (1981) Syndets zur Reinigung gesunder und erkrankter Haut. Ther der Gegenw 120: 1028–1045
2. Braun-Falco O (1983) Dermatologische Indikationen und Vorteile der Syndets. Ärztl Kosmetol 12: 354
3. Keining E (1959) Zur Frage der Reinigung gesunder und kranker Haut. Dermatol Wochenschr 140, 1245–1251
4. Klaschka F, Flasch CI, Weiland E (1985) Begleitende Behandlung von ekzematösen Erkrankungen mit pH-5-Eucerin®-Waschlotio. Ärztl Kosmetol 15: 35–38

5. Koch ME, Kligman AM (1983) Klinisch-experimentelle Untersuchungen zur Charakteristik von Seifen und Syndets. Pharmazeut Ztg 128: 963–968
6. Sachs L (1973) Angewandte Statistik – Planung und Auswertung. Methoden und Modelle. 4th ed. of Statistische Auswertungsmethoden. Springer, Berlin Heidelberg New York

Adjuvant Treatment with Synthetic Detergent Preparations in Atopic Dermatitis

W. Lechner

Background

Dermatologists are well aware that frequent washing will aggravate atopic dermatitis. On the other hand, it is felt that synthetic cleansers need not be avoided. The study described in this paper was undertaken in order to establish the efficacy of sebamed flüssig liquid cleanser in dermatitis.[1]

Material and Methods

Subjects

The sample was made up of 60 subjects (all females), of whom 30 had skin disorders (19 cases of atopic dermatitis, 9 cases of allergic contact dermatitis, 1 case of asteatotic eczema, 1 case of postscabetic dermatitis), and 30 had normal skins.

Equipment

The measurements of skin pH, skin surface lipids, and skin hydration were performed using an SMT-pH-90 pH meter, an SM 410 sebumeter, and a CM 420 corneometer, respectively (all equipment from Schwarzhaupt Medizintechnik GmbH, D-5000 Cologne 30).

The synthetic detergent cleanser used (sebamed flüssig, Sebapharma, Boppard, FRG), according to the manufacturers contains, amongst other ingredients, amino acids, nicotinic acid, nicotinamide, lactic acid, vitamin B6, vitamin H, and glycerol esters of essential unsaturated fatty acids; it is alkali-free, and has as pH of 5.5. For our study, a separate room was available for the entire day, with conditioning to keep the ambient temperature and humidity constant. The subjects were not under any physical or mental stress.

---

[1] This section is taken in part from Faulhaber G., Lechner W. (1986) Der Einfluß von sebamed flüssig Waschemulsion auf die ekzematöse Haut. Ärztliche Kosmetologie 16: 47–54, where a more thorough review of the subject will be found.

Trial Design

The dermatitis patients were asked to attend on two days. On each recording day, measurements were performed of skin pH, skin surface lipids, and hydration of the eczematous skin; the measuring sites were in the distal part of the right forearm, the distal part of the left forearm, and the middle of the forehead, using the most glabrous areas possible. The measuring sessions were between 0900 and 1000 hours, after a period of 24 hours during which no external dermatological or cosmetic agents had been allowed. The two recording days were at either end of an 8–10-day treatment period during which patients would receive their eczema therapy and, additionally, bathe the right forearm once a day, between 0900 and 1000 hours, for 10 minutes, in a solution of ca. 20 ml sebamed flssig Waschemulsion in 6 L water, at a temperature of 32 °C. After the treatment period, measurements were made between 0930 and 1430 hours, half an hour before the arm bath, and at intervals of half an hour, two hours, and four hours after the bathing of the right forearm.

The clinical course was assessed daily. The criteria used for monitoring the clinical effects of bathing the right forearm were redness of the skin, glistening, lichenification, scaling, excoriation, itching, and the patients' subjective impression. For purposes of comparison, the normal-skin controls were investigated in the same way as the dermatitis patients.

Results

In this paper, only results that proved statistically significant will be presented.
1. A comparison was made of the values, on Day 1, of pH, surface lipids, and hydration of the skin of both forearms and of the forehead of the dermatitis patients, with data from the same sites in the healthy controls.
Significance was tested using the Mann-Whitney U-test. Three differences were found to be significant ($p < 0.05$): The hydration of the skin of the left forearms and of the right forearms of the dermatitis patients was significantly lower ($p < 0.05$ on the left; $p < 0.01$ on the right) than the hydration of the left and right forearms, of the controls. The quantity of surface lipids on the forehead was significantly ($p < 0.001$) lower in the dermatitis patients than in the controls.
2. A comparison was made of the Day 1 values of pH, surface lipids, and hydration of the skin of the forearms and the forehead of the dermatitis patients, with the corresponding data measured after an 8–10-day treatment period, the measurements being performed half an hour before one forearm was bathed in sebamed flüssig liquid cleanser
Significance was tested using the Wilcoxon test. Four differences were found to be significant ($p < 0.05$): The values of skin hydration and surface lipids on both forearms of the dermatitis patients on the 2nd recording day 30 min before bathing the right forearm were significantly higher ($p < 0.05$) than the corresponding values obtained on Day 1.

3. A comparison was made of the data obtained from the forearms and the forehead of the dermatitis patients on the 2nd recording day, half an hour before, half an hour after, two hours after, and four hours after bathing of the right forearm.

   Significance was tested using the Wilcoxon test. Thirteen differences were found to be significant ($p < 0.05$), of which the following are of importance: The hydration of the eczematous skin of the right forearm was significantly ($p < 0.001$) higher 30 min after the forearm bath than it had been 30 min before bathing; it was significantly ($p < 0.05$) lower 2 hours after the forearm bath than 30 min after bathing; and significantly ($p < 0.05$) lower 4 hours after the forearm bath than at 30 min before and 30 min after bathing. The quantity of surface lipids of the eczematous right forearm skin was significantly ($p < 0.05$) lower 4 hours after the forearm bath than at 30 min after bathing.

   The pH of the eczematous right forearm skin was significantly ($p < 0.001$) higher 30 min after the forearm bath than at 30 min before bathing; it was significantly ($p < 0.01$) higher 2 hours after the forearm bath than at 30 min after bathing; significantly ($p < 0.05$) lower 4 hours after the forearm bath than at 2 hours after bathing; significantly ($p < 0.001$) higher 2 hours after the forearm bath than at 30 min before bathing; and significantly ($p < 0.001$) lower 4 hours after the forearm bath than at 30 min after bathing.

4. A comparison was made of all the data obtained from both forearms of the dermatitis patients.

   Significance was tested using the Mann-Whitney U-test. Three differences were found to be significant ($p < 0.05$): At 30 min, 2 hours, and 4 hours after the forearm bath, the pH of the eczematous right forearm skin was significantly ($p < 0.001$; $p < 0.01$; $p < 0.05$) higher than the pH of the eczematous left forearm skin.

Discussion

Unlike Finlay et al. [2], we found, in dermatitis patients, a reduced water content (as measured with the CM 420 corneometer) without a concomitant reduction in the quantity of surface lipids. We assume that, in dermatitis patients, the disturbance of keratinization (parakeratosis) also entails qualitative or functional epidermal lipid disturbances encouraging evaporation.

According to Blank and Shappirio [1], water, solvents, soap, and detergents can partly dissolve the Natural Moisturizing Factors (NMF) out of the stratum corneum, and thus produce a drying effect. However, in a separate analysis of the effects of the different agents, Gloor et al. [3] showed a drying effect of soap 10 minutes after application, whereas baseline hydration values had been restored within 10 minutes when synthetic detergents were used. In recording day measurements, a slight but statistically significant drying effect was found with detergents. However, the differences were not statistically significant when the right and left sides were compared. The same pattern was seen for surface lipids.

We did not find any decrease in the quantity of skin surface lipids, as measured with the SM 140 sebumeter. The measurements, at either end of the 8–10-day treatment period, carried out before the bathing of the right forearm, showed an increase in hydration and an increase in the amount of surface lipids on both sides. This effect may well be accounted for by the topical use of greasy agents. In the measurements on the recording day before and after forearm bathing, no difference in hydration or surface lipids was found between the right and left forearms.

If acid valences, which are responsible for pH, are removed from the skin by water or by surfactants, the pH of the skin surface will rise [5]. This pattern was demonstrated by our post-bathing forearm pH measurements with the SMT-pH-90 pH meter. The surprisingly large rise in pH after forearm bathing may be explained in terms of the great dilution of the synthetic detergent cleanser, and the intrinsic pH of water.

Like Finlay et al. [2] and Gloor et al. [4], we found in our study population that the measured data did not correlate with the clinical assessment. In 22 of the 30 patients, a beneficial effect of bathing in a synthetic cleanser solution was observed.

References

1. Blank IH, Shappirio EB (1955) The water content of the stratum corneum. Effect of previous contact with aqueous solutions of soaps and detergents. J Invest Dermatol 25: 391–401
2. Finley AY, Nicholls S, King CS, Mark R (1980) The dry non eczematous skin associated with atopic exzema. Brit Dermatol 102: 249–256
3. Gloor M, Hirsch G, Willebradt U (1981) On the use of infrared spectroscopy for the in vivo measurement of the water content of the horny layer after application of dermatological ointments. Arch Dermatol Res 271: 305–313
4. Gloor M, Heymann B, Stuhlert Th (1981) Infrared spectroscopic determination of the water content of the horny layer in healthy subjects and in persons suffering from atopic dermatitis. Arch Dermatol Res 271: 429–436
5. Tronnier H (1985) Seifen und Syndets in der Hautpflege und -therapie. Ärztl Kosmetol 15: 19–30

The Use of Synthetic Skin Cleansers in Neonates and Infants

F. Braun, Dorothea Lachmann, and H. Howanietz

There are several anatomical and functional aspects in which the skin of neonates and infants differs from adult skin: The epidermal attachment to the dermis is less adherent; the stratum corneum is more permeable; and melanin production is low. At birth, 80% of the hair follicles are in the resting state, and sweat is not produced until 24 to 48 hours after birth. Under the influence of maternal hormones, the sebaceous glands show increased activity in the neonatal period – a phenomenon that has been called the "miniature puberty of the newborn" – to begin a period of quiescence shortly afterwards that lasts until the onset of puberty [1]. However, it is not only in anatomical and functional respects that the skin of neonates and infants differs from adult skin. Physical and chemical properties specific to this very early age group have also been found. Thus, the skin pH of very young infants is alkaline [2], and the lipid layer contains only small amounts of free fatty acids [3].

In order to cater for this very special skin type, industry has come up with a wide range of baby skin cleansing products. In a previous study, we were able to show that, in infant skin, acidic pH synthetic detergent cleansers will cause less pH displacement after washing than will conventional soap [4].

This study was performed in order to monitor the pH as well as the lipid and hydration patterns of infant skin at defined intervals after washing with different agents – synthetic cleansers, alkaline soap, and plain tap water (as a control) – with analysis of the data obtained, and comparison of the results.

Subjects and Method

The study involved 40 infants aged 2 weeks to 14 months, who were required to have normal skin. The subjects were divided into 4 groups:

Group 1 = control group. These infants were washed with plain tap water
 (n = 10)
Group 2 = liquid synthetic detergent cleanser group (n = 10)
Group 3 = synthetic detergent bar group (n = 10)
Group 4 = alkaline soap group (n = 10)

The liquid synthetic cleanser used was a foam bath, Baby Sebamed-foam bath (pH 5.5); the synthetic cleanser bar was Baby Sebamed-Syndet bar (pH 5.5); and the alkaline soap was Baby Lux bar soap.

pH measurements were made with a flat membrane electrode (B232C) and a calomel reference electrode (K401) (Radiometer, Copenhagen) connected to a pH meter from the same firm.

Calibration and check calibrations were done before and after each run, in pH 7.00 phosphate buffer. During measurements, care was taken to ensure that the two electrodes were kept exactly 2 cm apart. The run was stopped after the pH had remained steady for 30 seconds. The skin lipid content was determined using a sebumeter (Schwarzhaupt, Cologne); and skin hydration was measured with a corneometer (Schwarzhaupt).

The following measuring sites were chosen: The gluteal region on the right, over the greater trochanter, and the skin over the manubrium of the sternum, as sites representative of non-exposed skin; and the dorsum of the right hand as well as the right cheek, as sites representative of exposed skin.

The statistical analysis was done using the Wilcoxon matched pairs test and the Mann-Whitney U-test. In order to answer the questions investigated in this study, we performed pre- and post-wash comparisons both within and between the groups, looking separately at the patterns in exposed and in non-exposed skin.

Results

The average age of the subjects (in months) was 3.5 in Group 1; 6.6 in Group 2; 4.8 in Group 3; and 4.7 in Group 4.

The mean pre-wash pH was 6.60, without any significant differences between the groups. After washing, skin surface pH values had become more alkaline in all groups, both at exposed and at non-exposed sites. However, the pre- to post-wash pH differences were statistically significant only when alkaline soap had been used (Group 4); in this group, these differences were found at the non-exposed sites only at 10 minutes after washing, and at the exposed sites at 10 minutes and at 30 minutes after washing (Fig. 1a, b).

Skin lipids were removed from the superficial skin level, in a statistically significant way, regardless of the washing agent used. The non-exposed site patterns of Groups 1, 2, and 3 were similar at 10 minutes after washing. Therefore, the comparison between the groups failed to show a statistically significant difference. The lipid loss was between 37 and 52%. However, in Group 4 the lipid loss at 10 minutes was 93%, which meant that it was significantly higher than the losses in the other groups. At 30 minutes, Groups 1–3 showed no major change, whereas in Group 4 restoration of skin lipids had decreased the lipid loss to 68%. At 60 minutes, restoration of skin lipids could be observed in all the groups; and at 120 minutes, Groups 1 and 2 had lipid levels that did not differ significantly from the pre-wash ones, while the difference was still 36% in Groups 3 and 4 (Fig. 2a).

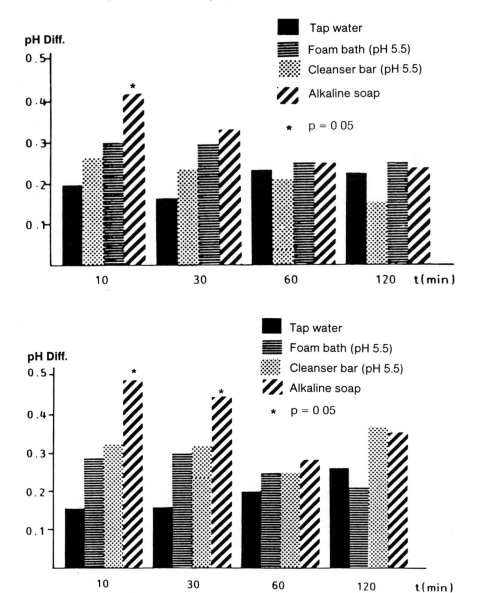

Fig. 1. Skin pH differences between pre-wash and 10, 30, 60, and 120 min post-wash (mean values): a) = non-exposed skin, b) = exposed skin
Group 1 (control group) = washing with tap water
Group 2 = washing with liquid synthetic cleanser (foam bath)
Group 3 = washing with cleanser bar
Group 4 = washing with alkaline soap
* Difference statistically significant at the 5 % level

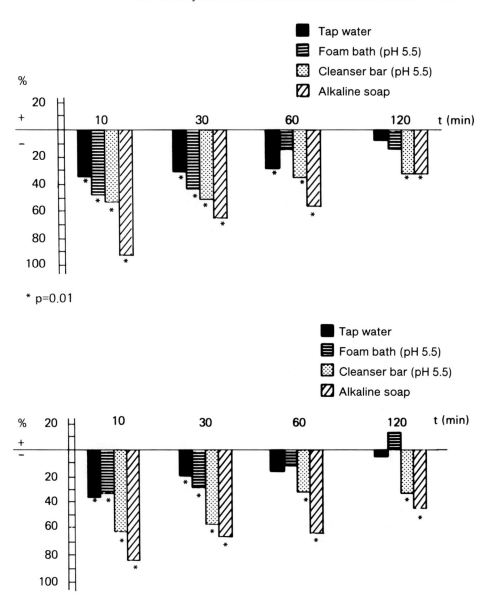

Fig. 2. Comparison of skin lipid content between pre-wash and 10, 30, 60, and 120 min post-wash. Decrease (−), increase (+) after washing, in % of pre-wash levels: a) = non-exposed skin, b) = exposed skin
Group 1 (control group) = washing with tap water
Group 2 = washing with liquid synthetic cleanser (foam bath)
Group 3 = washing with cleanser bar
Group 4 = washing with alkaline soap
* Difference statistically significant at the 1 % level

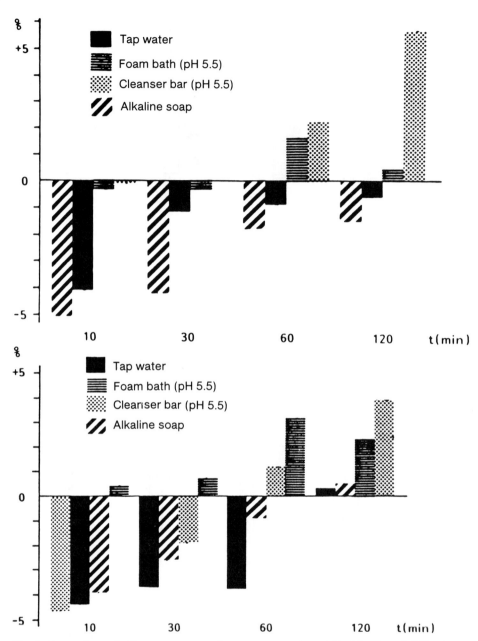

Fig. 3. Comparison of skin water content between pre-wash and 10, 30, 60, and 120 min post-wash. Decrease (−), increase (+) after washing, in % of pre-wash levels: a) = non-exposed skin, b) = exposed skin
Group 1 (control group) = washing with tap water
Group 2 = washing with liquid synthetic cleanser (foam bath)
Group 3 = washing with cleanser bar
Group 4 = washing with alkaline soap

At the exposed sites, the lipid loss from the skin surface at 10 minutes after washing was about the same in Groups 1 and 2 (31% and 36%, respectively); in Group 3, the loss was 62%; and in Group 4, 84%. Consequently, the comparison between the groups showed a statistically significant difference between Groups 1 and 2 on the one hand, and Groups 3 and 4 on the other hand, with a lipid loss in Group 4 that was significantly higher than in any of the other groups. At 30 minutes, restoration of skin lipids could be seen in all the groups, with markedly higher values than at the preceding measurement; and by 60 minutes after washing, Groups 1 and 2 were back to pre-wash lipid levels. However, as late as 120 minutes after washing, Groups 3 and 4 were still 32% and 43%, respectively, below pre-wash levels (Fig. 2b).

The water content went down, at the non-exposed sites, in Groups 1, 3, and 4; while remaining unchanged or even rising slightly above the pre-wash level in Group 2. The maximum water loss was 4.6%. In the statistical analysis of the data, no significant differences were found either in the comparison of the pre- and post-wash values or between the groups. The pattern was similar for the exposed sites: Groups 1 and 4 showed decreased hydration at 120 minutes; while there was virtually no change in Groups 2 and 3 out to 30 minutes after washing, followed by a rise to above pre-wash hydration levels. None of the differences found was statistically significant (Fig. 3a, b).

Summary

Plain tap water may be considered as an inert agent in skin cleanser studies; however, it acts as a solvent for chemical detergents, and was therefore chosen as a control. As our results show, liquid and solid (bar-type) synthetic detergent cleansers do not change the pH of the skin surface, while alkaline soap affects the acid mantle of the skin.

Skin lipids are removed from the superficial strata by all the agents, including plain tap water. The lipid loss at the non-exposed sites when using liquid or solid synthetic cleansers was the same as with plain tap water. At the exposed sites, more lipids were removed from the skin when the cleanser bar was used, as compared with plain tap water or the liquid cleanser formulation. Alkaline soap has the strongest defatting action (93% and 84%, respectively).

The hydration data do not show any statistically significant differences between the various agents; however, synthetic cleansers would once again appear to be beneficial. Since the post-wash differences observed were slight, larger studies, with more subjects per group, would have to be performed in order to obtain statistically significant information.

References

1. Solomon LM, Esterly NB (1970) Neonatal dermatology I. The newborn skin. J Pediatr 77: 888–894
2. Pantlischko M, Wildhalm J, Zweymüller E (1966) Einfluß der Pflege auf das Haut-pH der gesunden reifen Neugeborenen. Wien Klin Wochenschr 78: 665–669
3. Ramasastry P, Downing DT, Pochi PE, Strauss JS (1970) Chemical composition of human skin surface lipids from birth to puberty. J Invest Dermatol 54: 139–144
4. Braun F, Lachmann D, Zweymüller E (1986) Der Einfluß eines synthetischen Detergenz (Syndet) auf das pH der Haut von Säuglingen. Hautarzt 37: 329–334

Unwanted Effects of Synthetic Detergent Cleansers when Used in Normal or in Diseased Skin

Allergological Evaluation of Synthetic Skin Cleansers

J. Ring and R. Gollhausen

Background

Surfactants are contained in many products handled in everyday life (Table 1). Skin care products are usually listed among "Cosmetics" in international studies [1, 9, 16, 17, 22, 28, 34]. The risk index of cosmetics that derives from a large-scale FDA study shows surfactants in all the risk categories, from "high" (bath additives), through "medium" (soap), to "low" (shampoos) (Table 2). This scatter in the risk gradings is in itself a reason why general conclusions are difficult to draw.

Table 1. Products that contain surfactants

Laundry and dish washing products
Soaps (bar soap, liquid soap)
Shampoos
Bath additives
Other cosmetics; medicines

Surfactants may enter the body by different routes (ingestion, inhalation, injection, percutaneous absorption), and produce either local effects (in the skin or mucous membranes) or systemic ones.

Adverse Reaction Rates Following the Use of Surfactants

Without claiming to be exhaustive, Table 3 gives a list of publications on this subject, which shows a rate of adverse reactions following the application of surfactants of 0 to 12.6% [4–7, 29, 32].

A selection from seven major adverse reaction studies from Nater and de Groot shows soap to come sixth among the most frequent causative agents of adverse reactions to cosmetics (Table 4) [28].

Table 2. Risk grading of different cosmetics, from an FDA study ("Westat Report 1975") [4]

		Cosmetic units per experience
Depilatories Antiperspirants Hairspray Hair colours Face care Bath foam and oil	high	(<1000)
Make-up Lipstick Body talc Perfume Nail cosmetics Soap	medium	(1000–4000)
Shampoo Permanent wave Shaving aids Toothpaste Mouth freshener Hand and body lotion Foot cosmetics Sun cosmetics	low	(>4000)

Table 3. Adverse reactions to soap or soapless cleansers, in various studies (this list does not claim to be exhaustive)

%	Total (Subjects)	Author	Year
12.6	589	FDA study [6]	1975
12.0	626	Consumers' Association (UK) [7]	1979
9.5	698	US Dept. of Commerce [5]	1978
4.1	210	Romagnera et al. [32]	1983
3.7	8399	US Dept. of Commerce [6]	1975
0	96	Ngangu et al. [29]	1983

Table 4. The "Top 6" of adverse reactions-causing cosmetic products (from a selection from seven major international studies according to Nater and de Groot, 1985) [28]

1. Face care
2. Deodorant/antiperspirant
3. Eye makeup
4. Nail cosmetics
5. Hair colours
6. Soap

Mechanisms of Adverse Reactions to Surfactants

The majority of adverse reactions following the use of detergents may be assumed to be irritant in nature, with the surfactant causing the reaction. However, each individual case would have to be studied in order to establish whether the adverse experience was due to
– proper use of the product,
– improper use of the product, or
– an accident.

This more detailed assessment will obviously have a major impact on the side-effect profile of a substance. Improper use or accidents may be expected to result in toxic effects [8, 11, 16, 17, 28].

The other main group of adverse reactions is that of allergy, as a result of immunological sensitization [31]. Such reactions have been described for cosmetics that contain surfactants. In the majority of cases, the subjects concerned are allergic, not to the surfactant constituent of the soap or soapless cleanser, but to other ingredients, such as perfume, colouring agents, or metal salts (Table 5) [3, 14, 15, 21, 26, 33, 40, 41].

Table 5. Demonstrated contact allergies to soap constituents* (selection)

Perfume	Rothenborg and Hjorth [33]	(1968)
Colophony	Cooke and Kurwa [14]	(1972)
Mercury	Alomar et al. [3]	(1983)
Monosulfiram	Dick and Adams [15]	(1979)
Colouring (D&C Yellow No. 11)	Jordan [21]	(1981)
Colouring (D&C Yellow No. 11)	Weaver [41]	(1983)
Chromate	Mathias [26]	(1982)

* excluding photo-allergy

True immunological sensitization to the surfactant itself is rarer yet; however, anecdotal cases have been described (Table 6) [2, 10, 13, 23, 27, 35, 36, 37, 38].

One particularly interesting aspect is the possibility, suggested by several authors [12], of a surfactant exerting a combined effect – an irritant one, which may also facilitate sensitization to other foreign substances administered at the same time. Thus, enhanced penetration of chromate ions into the epidermis was found following the application of sodium lauryl sulphate [34]. In guinea pigs, Vinson and Choman [39] found an increased sensitization rate to nickel sulphate when sodium lauryl sulphate had been applied concurrently [39].

Kligman and Epstein observed an intensification of the allergic contact dermatitis reaction in volunteers, during the induction and challenge phases, when sodium lauryl sulphate had been used [22].

Table 6. Demonstrated contact allergies to surfactants

Triethanolamine	Thyresson et al. [36]	(1956)
Miranols	Verbov [38]	(1969)
Na-lauryl ether sulphate (+impurities)	Alchangan [2]	(1976)
Na-lauryl ether sulphate (+impurities)	Magnusson and Gilje [23]	(1973)
Na-lauryl ether sulphate (+impurities)	Sylvest et al. [35]	(1975)
Alkyl ethoxy sulphates (sultones)	Conner et al. [13]	(1975)
Lauryl dimethyl aminoxide	Muston et al. [27]	(1977)
Cocobetaine	Van Haute and Dooms-Goossens [37]	(1983)

However, Malten et al., who determined the nickel content of different detergents and performed threshold studies, came to the conclusion that the amounts of nickel contained in detergent products did not constitute a clinical nickel allergy hazard [25].

Clinical Investigations of Cases of Suspected Surfactant Allergy

Patients suspected of being allergic to a surfactant must be subjected to a detailed allergological investigation.

A comprehensive history must be obtained, establishing the chemical nature of the causative agents (including details on the manufacturer, batch number, etc.). Among the tests used, patch tests are of prime importance. Various types and modifications of patch tests have been evolved (Table 7). One important aspect is the distinction to be made between allergy on the one hand, and non-allergic (irritant) reactions on the other, by using appropriate test concentrations and by studying control populations [18, 19].

Table 7. Patch test modifications used in the allergological diagnosis of adverse reactions to surfactants

Open
Immediate reading
Conventional
Repeated
Photopatch
With stripping of stratum corneum
With surfactant
(starting at toxic concentrations, e. g. DNCB)
Dose-effect relationship
(test concentration, titration)
(finished detergent product; individual surfactants)
Test area
Contact-allergy time
Time of testing
(before, during, after exposure)

Table 8. Theoretical, animal experimental, and practical approaches to the allergological assessment of a proposed new surfactant

---

Theory (chemistry, toxicology, "allergo-toxicology")

In-vitro studies (?)

Animal experiments (e.g. guinea pigs, maximization test, etc.)

Volunteers
   (normal skins; atopics; contact allergy patients)
   (patch test; use tests)

Clinical and epidemiological studies
   Manufacturing personnel (laboratory; processing; handling)
   Users
     – prospective monitoring
     – spontaneous experience reports
       (proper use; improper use; accidents)

Case reports

In order to establish the nature of the contact dermatitis, provocative use tests and repeated open application tests (ROAT) have been described for cosmetics (Table 8) [24].

Allergy Risks of New Detergents

Any newly developed agent will be judged in the light of theoretical information on its chemical structure, as well as by animal experiments (e.g. guinea pig models, etc.). In addition, trials will be carried out in volunteers, using patch tests or use tests. There will also be clinical and epidemiological studies once the product is on the market, and case reports of any adverse reactions encountered will be collected (Table 8) [30, 31].

The assessment of a particular product may be far from easy, as was demonstrated by the case of a new washing powder introduced in Britain some years ago [20, 42]. Unlike the earlier formula, the new product contained enzymes, and soon there were reports of "skin complaints." It was decided to do skin tests in 255 subjects from the London area. All the prick and patch tests proved negative. Only one patch test showed a reaction to the standard perfume, and one to nickel sulphate. A user test was arranged, in which the subjects were made to wear, for 5 days, vests washed in the new formula washing powder and in a control powder, respectively. Two skin reactions were seen following washing with the enzyme-containing powder, and three following washing with the non-enzyme control. The authors concluded that there was no proven relationship between the dermatoses observed and the new formula washing powder [42].

Conclusions

In the allergological assessment of detergents, a strict distinction must be made between the different types of use and – above all – the different circumstances preceding the adverse reactions reported. It would be desirable for candidate substances to be allergologically screened, so as to exclude potential sensitizers from the start; a wide range of models (including in-vitro studies) could and should be used in order to obtain as much information as possible.

Summary

Adverse reactions to soaps or soapless cleansers are usually irritant in nature. True allergy is rare, and is usually caused by such ingredients as perfume, colouring agents, or metal salts. Contact allergy to pure surfactants is rarer yet, but not totally unknown. The investigation of adverse reactions attributed to a synthetic detergent cleanser requires careful examination, including various patch tests. Comparisons should also be performed with suitable control groups, in order to distinguish allergic reactions from irritant ones. Whether a newly developed substance will act as a sensitizer is very much more difficult to assess. Information may be derived from a theoretical knowledge of the chemical structure and composition of the substance concerned, as well as from animal models, which are particularly informative in this respect. It would be desirable to have in-vitro methods for this assessment. Preclinical studies in volunteers, using patch tests and user tests, and post-marketing product monitoring are equally important in the overall strategy of the allergological assessment of a cleanser.

References

1. Adam WE, Neumann K (1980) Konstitution und Eigenschaften von Tensiden. Fette, Seifen, Anstrichmittel 83: 367–370
2. Alchangyan LV (1976) Selisskii. Khim Promst (Moscow) 8: 635
3. Alomar A, Camarasa IG, Barnadas M (1983) Addison's disease and contact dermatitis from mercury in a soap. Contact Dermatitis 9: 76–79
4. Anonymous. Tabulation of Cosmetic Product Experience Report. (Jan. 1974–June 1975). Food & Drug Administration, Division of Cosmetic Technology, Washington DC, USA, 200 C'street SW
5. –. Cosmetic-related injuries: A MODS study of NEISS. July 1st 1977 to June 30th 1978. National Technical Information Service, US Department of Commerce, Springfield, 22161, USA
6. –. An investigation of Consumers perception of adverse reactions to cosmetics products. (PB-242 480) Westat Inc. Prepared for Food and Drug Administration. June 1975. National Technical Information US Department of Commerce, Springfield, 22161, USA
7. –. Reactions of the skin to cosmetic and toiletry products (1979). Consumers' Association, 14 Buckingham Street. London WC2

8. Baer RL, Rosenthal SA (1954) The germicidal action in human skin of soap containing tetramethylthiuram disulfide. J Invest Dermatol 23: 193–211
9. Bartnik F, Künstler K (1986) Biological effects, toxicology and human safety. In: Falbe J (ed) Surfactants in consumer products. Springer, Berlin Heidelberg New York, pp 475–503
10. Blank IH (1956) Allergie hypersensitivity to an antiseptic soap. J Amer Med Ass 160: 1225–1226
11. Borelli S, Manok M (1961) Ergebnisse von Untersuchungen bei Berufsanfängern im Friseurgewerbe. Dermatosen Bcruf Umw 9: 271–274
12. Calnan CD (1964) The climate of contact dermatitis. Acta Derm Venereol (Stockh) 44: 33–43
13. Conner DS (1977) Identification of certain sultones as the sensitizers in an alkyl ethoxy sulfate. Fette, Seifen, Anstrichmittel 77: 25–29
14. Cooke MA, Kurva AR (1975) Colophony sensitivity. Contact Dermatitis 1: 192–193
15. Dick DC, Adams RH (1979) Allergic contact dermatitis from monosulfiram (Tetmosol) soap. Contact Dermatitis 5: 199–201
16. Estrin NF (ed) (1984) The cosmetic industry. Scientific and regulatory foundations. Marcel Dekker, New York
17. Fiedler HP, Umbach W (1986) Cosmetics and toiletries. In: Falbe J (ed) Surfactants in consumer products. Springer, Berlin Heidelberg New York, pp 352–397
18. Frosch PJ, Kligman AM (1979) The soap chamber test. A new method for assessing the irritancy of soaps. J Amer Acad Dermatol 1: 35–41
19. Gollhausen R, Kligman AM (1985) Human assay for identifiying substances which induce non-allergic contact uriticaria: the NICU-test. Contact Dermatitis 13: 98–106
20. Jensen ME (1970) Severe dermatitis and "biological" detergents. Brit Med J 1: 299–304
21. Jordan WP Jr (1981) Contact dermatitis from D & C yellow 11 dye in a toilet bar soap. J Amer Acad Derm 4: 613–615
22. Kligman AM, Epstein W (1975) Updating the maximization test for identifying contact allergens. Contact Dermatitis 1: 231–239
23. Magnusson B, Gilie O (1973) Allergic contact dermatitis from a dishwashing liquid containing lauryl ether sulphate. Acta Derm Venereol (Stockh) 53: 136–149
24. Maibach HI, Akerson JM, Marzulli FN, Wenninger J, Greif M, Hjorth N, Andersen KE, Wilkinson DS (1980) Test concentrations and vehicles for dermathological testing of cosmetic ingredients. Contact Dermatitis 6: 369–379
25. Malten KE, Schutter K, von Senden KG, Spruit D (1969) Nickel sensitization and detergents. Acta Derm Venereol (Stockh) 49: 10–13
26. Mathias CGT (1982) Pigmented cosmetic dermatitis from contact allergy to a toilet soap containing chromium. Contact Dermatitis 8: 29–33
27. Muston HL, BHoss JM, Summerly R (1977) Dermatitis from Ammonyx LO, constituent of surgical scrub. Contact Dermatitis 3: 347–350
28. Nater JP, de Groot AC, Liem DH (eds) (1985) Unwanted effects of cosmetics and drugs used in dermatology. 2nd ed. Elsevier, Amsterdam
29. Ngangu Z, Samsoen M, Foussereau J (1983) Einige Aspekte zur Kosmetika-Allergie in Straßburg. Dermatosen Beruf Umw 31: 126–130
30. Ring J, Fröhlich HH (1985) Wirkstoffe in der Dermatologie. 2nd ed. Springer, Berlin
31. Ring J (1988) Angewandte Allergologie, 2nd ed. MMV-Vieweg, München
32. Romaguera C, Camarasa JMG, Alomar A, Grimalt F (1983) Patch tests with allergens related to cosmetics. Contact Dermatitis 9: 167–170
33. Rothenborg HW, Hjorth N (1968) Allergy to perfumes from toilet soaps and detergents in patients with dermatitis. Arch Dermatol 97: 417–421
34. Schwarz E (1962) Symp Dermatol 1: 250
35. Sylvest B, Hjorth N, Magnusson B (1975) Lauryl ether sulphate dermatitis in Denmark. Contact Dermatitis 1: 359–364
36. Thyresson N, Lodin A, Nilzen A (1956) Eczema of the hands due to triethanolamine in cosmetic hand lotions for housewives. Acta Derm Venereol (Stockh) 36: 355–359

37. Van Haute N, Dooms-Goossens A (1983) Shampoo dermatitis due to cocobetaine and soudium lauryl ether sulphate. Contact Dermatitis 9: 169–174
38. Verbov JL (1969) Contact dermatitis from Miranols. Trans St John's Hosp Derm Soc (Lond) 55: 192–197
39. Vinson LJ, Choman BR (1960) J Soc Cosmet Chem 11: 127
40. Walker AP, Ashforth GK, Davies RE, Newman EA, Ritz HL (1973) Some characteristics of the sensitizer in alkyl ethoxy sulphate. Acta Derm Venereol (Stockh) 43: 141–144
41. Weasver JE (1983) Dose respnse relationships in delayed hypersensitivity to quinoline dyes. Contact Dermatitis 9: 309–312
42. White IR, Lewis J, Alami AE (1985) Possible adverse reactions to an enzyme containing washing powder. Contact Dermatitis 13: 175–180

Factors Involved in the Irritancy Testing of Synthetic Cleanser Constituents

R. Gollhausen

Introduction

The use of soap or synthetic cleansers for skin care will only exceptionally result in contact allergy [62]. In everyday use, the much more relevant – and comparatively frequent – phenomenon is the irritant effect of detergents on the skin, which is, of course, closely related to the detersive action the product is intended to provide [10, 19, 54–56, 61, 68]. Whereas in the investigation of a possible contact allergy, the main question is "What?" rather than "How much?" – since the patient either is or is not allergic to, say, lanolin alcohols -, irritant dermatitis is chiefly a question of "How much?" – which, in the case of cleansers, boils down to a question of how much cleansing the skin can stand without getting damaged. (Table 1) [12, 21, 51, 58].

Table 1. Principal differences between contact allergy and irritant dermatitis

Contact allergy	Irritant dermatitis
e.g. by lanolin alcohols	e.g. by soda lye
– requires a sensitization phase	– possible on first contact
– usually an exceptional event	– could, in principle, affect anyone
– question of "What?"	– question of "How much?"
– diagnosed from patch tests	– diagnostic tests ?
– uniform pathogenetic mechanism	– diverse pathogenetic mechanisms

The diagnosis of allergy relies upon techniques (patch tests for contact allergies; maximization test for sensitization potential) that are much better established than the tests used in irritancy testing [33, 50]. Although great efforts have been made, dermatologists, to date, do not have a reliable, universal technique – along the lines of the chest physician's lung function tests – to enable them to detect sensitive skin [5, 18, 51].

This deficiency is due to the fact that skin function is described in terms of a number of very different parameters that have not, as yet, been clearly defined (Table 2) [3, 7, 17, 18, 63, 65]. Thus "dry skin" – to mention but one feature – contains many parameters, some of which are unknown: Apart from skin lipids,

Table 2. Parameters of interest in irritancy testing (selection)

- Clinical features (redness, scaling, cracks, etc.)
- Symptoms (pain, itching, tension)
- Skin blood flow
- pH
- Alkali neutralization time, alkali resistance
- Roughness
- Skin elasticity
- Surface pattern
- Surface lipids
- Surface water content
- Water loss
- Heat loss
- Electrical conductivity

there are such quantities as hydration, roughness, subclinical signs of inflammation, and several other aspects which all come under this heading [39, 52, 57, 67].

It obviously follows that, in the testing of synthetic cleanser constituents, a host of factors have to be borne in mind; Table 3 mentions but a few [25, 51].

Skin Type

Any cosmetic or medicinal skin care agent must be compatible with the skin type of the user. Thus, a defatting action is desirable in a patient with seborrhoea, but would be contra-indicated in someone with dry skin. It has been stated that

Table 3. Factors examined in irritancy testing

- Skin type
- Age, sex, race
- Chronobiological rhythms
- Medication; concomitant disease
- Neurological factors
- Dose and concentration
- Duration and frequency of exposure
- Temperature
- Mechanical factors
- Occlusion
- Invisible pre-existing skin lesions
- Exposed surface area
- Site
- Penetration
- pH
- Relative humidity; climate
- Skin hyperreactivity ("status eczematicus")
- Vehicle
- Other ingredients

subjects with a dry skin prefer alkaline soaps, whereas seborrhoeic subjects prefer synthetic cleansers [58, 68]. Consequently, the intended skin type should be taken into account in the prospective testing of synthetic cleansers, with proper definition and selection of the study groups. Since, as a rule, irritancy studies are performed only to establish the lower limit of toxicity, it would be useful to have preliminary studies in which subjects with sensitive skins would be exposed to comparable irritants. This approach could help to reduce the great scatter normally observed in irritancy testing [21–23, 35, 45, 60].

Selection of Subjects

In the selection of subjects, consideration must be given to such factors as age, sex, race, medication, concomitant disease, neurological factors, chronobiological rhythms, etc. Older subjects appear to be less prone to acute irritation by certain substances. However, older subjects tend to suffer from conditions such as asteatotic eczema, which may be due to less efficient regeneration mechanisms [4, 5, 13, 27, 29, 36, 44, 45, 51, 52, 64].

In order further to reduce scatter and to facilitate comparability, intra-individual tests should be performed. However, irritancy tests will once again produce more variation than will allergy tests. In our own, previously unpublished, studies we were able to confirm the results obtained by Dahl et al. [14], who also found much greater variation in the response to irritants (not only sodium lauryl sulphate) than in the response to allergens, although, even with allergens, one and the same individual may produce different skin reactions [33, 40].

Type of Test

The quantity and concentration of the agent used, as well as the duration and frequency of exposure are of critical importance in the performance of tests. Often the actual product is improperly used in everyday life: too much of a cleanser or too strong a cleanser may be used; washing may be unduly prolonged; the water may be too hot. All of these factors would mean that even a mild cleanser may be found to be irritating. Indeed, if used too hot and for too long, plain water would produce irritation. Synthetic detergents are powerful cleansers and, as a result, often have a higher irritancy potential than soap. They therefore should be used more sparingly. These considerations are of vital importance in the testing and the use of synthetic cleansers, as shown by the discussion in the literature on the Duhring chamber test [9–11, 21, 38, 41, 60]. Irritation may also be caused by mechanical stress during washing, such as friction, pressure, or shear; by the substantivity of the product; and by the occlusion (a feature of chamber tests), which causes swelling of the stratum corneum, thereby greatly enhancing the irritancy potential [24, 30, 51, 61]. The result will also be affected by the size of the test area. If the area is too small, the irritant effect may appear to be less [18, 51].

Cumulative Insult

Invisible pre-existing skin lesions can affect the results in a major way [12, 51]. Since, in everyday life, subclinical skin damage is a frequent occurrence, and since even overtly diseased skin has to be cleansed, synthetic detergent cleansers should be tested, not only on intact skin, but also on skin bearing standardized lesions [19, 20, 41].

It is also vital that the test substances should be applied repeatedly, in order to provide at least some rough and ready simulation of the pathogenesis of cumulative insult dermatitis. Lesions that are not visible initially, and a reduced regeneration potential, will show up as the test is repeated; also, the rinsability of the cleanser may change, since, as the skin becomes dry and rough, it will not only trap dirt more easily, but also retain the cleanser, making it more difficult to remove [21, 22, 49, 52].

Site

There are major differences between the various skin regions in terms, not only of penetration of substances, but of response to irritants. Thus it is an established clinical fact that higher cortisone or anthralin concentrations are tolerated by the scalp than in the axilla, even though the penetration of hydrocortisone, for instance, is almost the same in the scalp and in the axilla [16, 24]. Thus, the penetration of a substance is insufficient to characterize its irritancy potential [51, 59].

pH

Some authors have claimed pH to be a major factor in determining the irritancy potential of cleansers. However, the results adduced in support of this claim are not wholly conclusive, and – except for results obtained at extreme pH ranges – the evidence provided so far would not appear to prove that pH has a major influence on the irritancy potential of a substance [8, 26, 37, 43, 53–56, 61, 64, 66, 68, 70, 72].

Season

More irritation is produced in winter, probably as a result of the increased dryness of the skin resulting from lower relative humidity. This is why an agent found to be non-irritating in the summer may turn out to be more adverse when used during the winter months. Ultraviolet light protects against irritants, by causing skin thickening as well as by other mechanisms [1, 15, 28, 29, 31, 32, 46].

Skin Hyperreactivity

Generalized non-specific hyperreactivity of the skin ("status eczematicus"; "angry back") may occur in repeated testing in volunteers, even if the initial test site is no longer visibly irritated. Calnan [12] has described a classical example of this phenomenon: In company personnel that had undergone frequent testing, von Hamm and Mallette found two test substances to be severely irritating and moderately sensitizing; when the same agents were tested in "virgin" students, they were found to be completely safe.

Vehicle

The vehicle in which the test substance is administered is of crucial importance. Soaps and synthetic cleansers certainly are more irritant when applied with water as a vehicle than when administered in white soft paraffin. Obviously, tests should be done, not only on the individual ingredients, but on the fully formulated product, since there are many possible interactions [51, 58, 61].

In-vitro, Animal, and Human Studies

Since irritancy testing in humans is a complex subject, the question arises whether in-vitro studies and animal models could not be used instead (Table 4) [3, 38, 63]. However, such tests can only be used to guide subsequent human trials, and cannot be expected to provide the detailed information required. In-vitro and animal studies (especially the Draize test) also suffer from considerable variation, which means that differences have to be very pronounced in order to show statistical significance [38]. As Adam and Neumann state, "The customary Draize test fails to show differences in mucous membrane irritancy between fatty alcohol sulphates with different cations, and ether sulphates. This makes the many claims of product superiority in the manufacturers' data sheets scientifically untenable." [2].

Thus, in order to obtain valid information, testing will have to be done in humans, taking into account the factors listed above (Table 4) [3, 19–22, 41, 60]. Wherever possible, several techniques should be combined, and the irritancy potential should be related to the cleansing potential of the product concerned. However, it is difficult to standardize detergency testing in human subjects, since many individual factors, some of which have been discussed under the heading of irritancy testing, will affect the situation (Table 5) [10, 63, 66]. The target group (intended user skin type) should be specified.

Table 4. Irritancy testing of detergents (selection)

a) *In vitro*
– Zein test
– Saccharase enzyme inhibition test
– Haemolysis test
– Release of sulphhydril groups
– Hydration of isolated porcine epidermis

b) *Animal models*
– Draize test
– Intracutaneous test
– Repeated open application
– Chamber test
– Vermeer's washing simulator

c) *Human procedures*
– Simple chamber test
– Frosch and Kligman's detergent test
– Scarification chamber test
– Wound healing test after formic acid application
– Wash test (antecubital fossa, face)

Non-invasive Techniques

Modern instruments such as the evaporimeter, the laser dual flow meter, and others have made it possible to obtain quantitative and validable information on individual skin sensitivity parameters. One major advance has come from the fact that it is now possible to detect skin irritation at a very early stage, when it may be barely perceptible on clinical examination. This early detection may be crucial to the testing of synthetic cleansers, and vital in the investigation and diagnosis of cumulative insult dermatitis. By now, it has become possible to distinguish, through objective measurements, between the pre- and post-treatment patterns of patients with atopic dermatitis, and between atopics with sensitive skins and healthy volunteers with normal skins. However, even these techniques are not free from variation (which may be considerable) and from inconsistency of results. Thus, benzalkonium chloride, while causing visible skin irritation, will not produce a major and measurable change in TEWL [6, 7, 25, 28, 29, 32, 34, 36, 37, 43–45, 48, 49, 64, 69–73].

Table 5. Detergency testing of detergents (selection)

– Standard washing of woollen swatches
– Degreasing of woollen yarn
– Degreasing test according to Würbach
– Wash test according to Tronnier
– Greiter's skin washing simulator

Conclusion

It will be necessary to produce new test methods, based upon a critical evaluation and consideration of all the factors involved in the testing of synthetic cleansers.

References

1. Abe T, Mayuzimi J, Kikuchi N, Arai S (1980) Seasonal variations in skin temperature, skin pH, evaporative water loss and skin surface lipid values on human skin. Chem Pharm Bull 28: 387–392
2. Adam WE, Neumann K (1980) Konstitution und Eigenschaften von Tensiden. Fette, Seifen, Anstrichmittel 82: 367–370
3. Bartnik F, Künstler K (1986) Biological effects, toxicology and human safety. In: Falbe J (ed): Surfactants in consumer products. Springer, Berlin Heidelberg New York, 475–503
4. Berardesca E, Maibach HI (1988) Racial differences in sodium lauryl sulphate induced cutaneous irritation: black and white. Contact Derm 18: 65–70
5. Björnberg A (1968) Skin reactions to primary irritants in patients with hand eczema. Isacsons, Göteborg
6. Blanken R, van der Valk PGM, Nater JP (1986) Laser doppler flowmetry in the investigation of irritant compounds of the human skin. Determatosen 34: 5–9
7. Blichmann CW, Serup J (1988) Assessment of skin moisture. Measurement of electrical conductance, capacitance and transepidermal water loss. Acta Derm Venereol 68: 284–290
8. Braun F, Lachmann D, Zweymüller E (1986) Der Einfluß eines synthetischen Detergens (Syndet) auf das pH der Haut von Säuglingen. Hautarzt 37: 329–334
9. Braun-Falco O (1984) Letter to the editor. Tests am Menschen. Ärztl Kosmetol 14: 153–156
10. Braun-Falco O (1988) Hautreinigung bei atopischem Ekzem (Neurodermitis diffusa, endogenes Ekzem). Ärztl Kosmetol 18: 276–278
11. Braun-Falco O, Heilgemeier GP (1981) Syndets zur Reinigung gesunder und erkrankter Haut. Ther Gegenw 120: 1028–1045
12. Calnan CD (1964) The climate of contact dermatitis. Acta Derm Venereol 44: 33–43
13. Coenraads PJ, Bleumink E, Nater JP (1975) Susceptibility to primary irritants. Age dependence and relation to contact allergie reactions. Contact Derm 1: 377–381
14. Dahl MV, Pass F, Trancik RJ (1984) Sodium lauryl sulfate irritant patch tests. II. Variations of test responses among subjects and comparison to variation of allergic responses elicited by Toxicodendron extract. J Am Acad Dermatol 11: 474–477
15. Enders F, Gollhausen R, Kligman AM, Przybilla B (1988) Jahreszeitliche Einflüsse auf die Hautreaktivität. Zbl Haut 154: 631
16. Feldmann RJ, Maibach HI (1967) Regional variation in percutaneous penetration of 14-C-cortisol in man. J Invest Dermatol 48: 181–186
17. Fiedler HP, Umbach W (1986) Cosmetics and toiletries. In: Falbe J (ed) Surfactants in consumer products. Springer, Berlin Heidelberg New York, 352–397
18. Frosch PJ (1981) Die empfindliche Haut. Methoden zur Erkennung der Riskofaktoren für Hautreizungen durch chemische Irritantien. Habilitationsschrift (postdoctoral thesis). Hautklinik der Westfälischen Wilhelms-Universität Münster
19. Frosch PJ, Klingman AM (1982) Recognition of chemically vulnerable and delicate skin. Chapter 36 in: Frost P, Horwitz SN (Eds): Principles of cosmetics for the dermatologist. C V Mosby Company, St. Louis Toronto London

20. Frosch PJ (1982) Irritancy of soaps and detergent bars. Chapter 1 in: Frost P, Horwitz SN (Eds) Principles of cosmetics for the dermatologist. C V Mosby Company, St. Louis Toronto London, 5–12
21. Frosch PJ (1983) Tests am Menschen. Testmodelle für Hautirritation am Menschen. Ärztl Kosmetol 13: 397–406
22. Frosch PJ, Kligman AM (1979) The soap chamber test. A new method for assessing the irritancy of soaps. J Am Acad Dermatol 1: 35–41
23. Frosch PJ, Kligman AM (1977) A method for appraising the stinging capacity of topically applied substances. J Soc Cosmet Chem 28: 197–209
24. Gloor M (1982) Pharmakologie dermatologischer Externa. Springer, Berlin Heidelberg New York
25. Gloor M, Wagner L (1985) Nichtimmunologische Funktionsstörungen der Haut beim Neurodermitiker. Zbl Haut 150: 505–509
26. Gloor M, Scheer T (1989) In-vivo-Regulation der Honrschichtfeuchtigkeit. Ärztl Kosmetol 19: 31–40
27. Goh GL, Chia SE (1988) Skin irritability to sodium lauryl sulphate – as measured by skin water loss – by sex and race. Clin Exper Dermatol 13: 16–19
28. Gollhausen R, Göttsberger K, Winter H, Przybilla B, Ring J (1988) The cutaneous blood flow as a new marker of skin sensitivity to UV-B. Evaluation in patients with atopic eczema and in controls. J Invest Dermatol 91: 385
29. Gollhausen R, Klutke U, Przybilla B, Ring J (1989) The cutaneous blood flow slope (CBFS) as a marker of skin sensitivity to UV-light. J Invest Dermatol 92: 435
30. Gollhausen R, Kligman AM (1985) Effects of Pressure on Contact Dermatitis. Amer J Ind Med 8: 323–328
31. Gollhausen R, Kaidbey K, Schlechter N (1985) UV suppression of mast cell-mediated whealing in human skin. Photodermatology 2: 58–67
32. Gollhausen R, Göttsberger K, Winter H, Przybilla B, Ring J (1987) Skin sensivity in atopic eczema (AE) before and after UVA phototherapy – evaluaton by visual assessment, evaporimeter and laser doppler flowmeter. J Invest Dermatol 89: 319
33. Gollhausen R, Przybilla B, Ring J (1989) Reproducibility of patch testing. J Am Acad Dermatol 21: 1196–1202
34. Gollhausen R, Göttsberger K, Winter H, Przybilla B, Ruzieka T, Ring J (1988) Skin sensitivity in patients with atopic eczema and normals – evaluation by visual assessment, evaporimeter and laser doppler flowmeter. J Invest Dermatol 90: 241
35. Gollhausen R, Kligman AM (1985) Human assay for identifying substances which induce non-allergic contact urticaria: the NICU-test. Contact Derm 13: 98–106
36. Guy RH, Tur E, Bjerke S, Maibach HI (1985) Are there age and racial differences to methyl nicotinate-induced vasodilatation in human skin. J Am Acad Dermatol 12: 1001–1006
37. Hassing JH, Natr JP, Bleumink E (1982) Irritancy of low concentrations of soap and synthetic detergents as measured by skin water loss. Dermatologica 164: 314–321
38. Kästner W, Frosch PJ (1981) Hautirritationen verschiedener anionaktiver Tenside im Duhring-Kammer-Test am Menschen im Vergleich zu in-vitro- und tierexperimentellen Methoden. Fette, Seifen, Anstrichmittel 83: 33–46
39. Kligman AM, Lavker RM, Grove GL, Studemayer TJ (1982) Some aspects of dry skin and its treatment. In: Kligman AM, Leyden JJ (eds) Safety and efficacy of topical drugs and cosmetics. Grune & Straton, New York, 221–238
40. Kligman AM, Gollhausen R (1986) The "angry back"; a new concept or old confusion? Br J Dermatol 115, Suppl 31: 93–100
41. Koch E, Frenk E, Ligman AM (1983) Experimentelle und klinische Untersuchungen auf Hautirritation durch Syndets. Ärztl Kosmetol 13: 11–20
42. Korting HC, Kober M, Mueller M, Braun-Falco O (1987) Influence of repeated washings with soap and synthetic detergents on pH and resident flora of the skin of forehead and forearm. Acta Derm Venereol (Stockh) 67: 41–47
43. Lammintausta K, Maibach HI, Wilson D (1987) Human cutaneous irritation: induced hyporeactivity. Contact Derm 17: 193–198

44. Lammintausta K, Maibach HI, Wilson D (1987) Irritant reactivity in males and females. Contact Derm 17: 276–280
45. Lammintausta K, Maibach HI (1988) Exogenous and endogenous factors in skin irritation. Int J Dermatol 27: 213–222
46. Lehmann P, Helbig S, Hölzle E, Plewig G (1988) Bestrahlung mit UV-A oder UV-B wirkt protektiv gegenüber Irritantien. Zbl Haut 154: 686–692
47. Lejman E, Stoudemayer T, Grove G, Kligman AM (1984) Age differences in poison ivy dermatitis. Contact Derm 11: 163–167
48. Maibach HI, Bronaugh R, Guy R, Turr E, Wilson D, Jacques WS, Chaing D (1984) Noninvasive techniques for determining skin function. In: Drill VA (ed) Cutaneous Toxicology. Raven Press, New York
49. Malten KE, den Arend JACJ (1985) Irritant contact dermatitis. Traumiterative and cumulative impairment by cosmetics, climate, and other daily loads. Dermatosen 33: 125–132
50. Marzulli FN, Maibach HI (1986) Contact allergy: predictive testing in humans. In: Marzulli FN, Maibach HI (eds) Dermatoxicology. Hemisphere Publishing Corporation, Washington 319–340
51. Mathias CGT (1986) Clinical and experimental aspects of cutaneous irritation. In: Marzulli FN, Maibach HI (eds) Dermatoxicology. Hemisphere Publishing Corporation, Washington, 173–189
52. Meinhof W (1970) Degenerativ-toxische und Exsiccationsschäden der Haut. In: Braun-Falco O, Bandmann HJ (eds) Fortschritte der praktischen Dermatologie und Venerologie. Springer, Berlin, Vol 6: 93–102
53. Murahata RI, Toton-Quinn R, Finkey MB (1988) Effect of pH on the production of irritation in a chamber irritation test. J Am Acad Dermatol 18: 62–66
54. Anon. (1987) Test Waschlotionen (Syndets): Seifenfrei und etwas teurer,. Stiftung Warentest, Test 4: 364–367
55. Anon. (1989) Test Haarshampoo. Nicht alle gut für den Kopf. Stiftung Warentest, Test 2: 177–181
56. Anon. (1989) Test Duschbäder. Manche gehen an die Haut. Stiftung Warentest, Test 3: 234–238
57. Pierard GE (1987) What does "dry skin" mean? Int J Dermatol 26: 167–168
58. Proksch E (1986) Anforderungen des Dermatologen an Badepräparate. Ärztl Kosmetol 16: 130–134
59. Prottey C, Ferguson T (1975) Factors which determine the skin irritation potential of soaps and detergents. J Soc Cosmet Chem 26: 29–46
60. Puschmann M, Meyer-Rohn J (1983) Hautverträglichkeitsnachweis neuartiger Syndetpräparate auf der Basis von Äthersulfaten, Amidobetainen, Sulfosuccinaten und Isäthionaten. Ärztl Kosmetol 13: 225–234
61. Raab W (1987) Zur Reinigung gesunder und kranker Haut. Ärztl Kosmetol 17: 354–359
62. Ring J, Gollhausen R (1990) Allergologische Bewertung von Syndets zur Hautreinigung. In: Braun-Falco O, Korting HC (eds) (1990) Hautreinigung mit Syndets pp. 181–188. Springer, Berlin Heidelberg
63. Schrader KH (1987) Die Bedeutung der Reinigung im Bereich der Kosmetik: In: Greiter F (ed) Akutelle Technologien in der Kosmetik. Hüthig, Heidelberg, 115–117
64. Thune P, Nilsen T, Hanstad K, Gustavsen T, Lövig Dahl H (1988) The water barrier function of the skin in relation to the water content of stratum corneum. pH and skin lipids. Acta Derm Venereol (Stockh) 68: 277–283
65. Tronnier H (1984) Meßmethoden an der Haut zur Ermittlung der Wirkung kosmetischer Präparate. Parfümerie und Kosmetik 65: 454–466
66. Tronnier H (1985) Seifen und Syndets in der Hautpflege und -therapie. Ärztl Kosmetol 15: 19–30
67. Uehara M (1986) Dry skin (sebostasis) and inflammation: heterogencity of "dry skin" in atopic dermatitis. In: Ring J (ed) New Trends in Allergy II. Springer, Berlin Heidelberg New York

68. Ummenhofer B (1982) Praktische berufsdermatologische Aspekte der Hautreinigung. Zbl Haut Geschl-Kr 147: 379–449
69. Van der Valk PGM, Nater JP, Bleumink E (1984) Skin irritancy of surfactants as assessed by water vapor loss measurements. J Invest Dermatol 82: 291–293
70. Van der Valk PGM, Nater JP, Bleumink E (1985) Vulnerability of the skin to surfactants in different groups of eczema patients and controls as measured by water vapour loss. Clin Exper Dermatol 10: 185–193
71. Van der Valk PGM, Nater JP, Bleumink E (1985) The influence of low concentrations of irritants on skin barrier function as determined by water vapour loss. Dermatosen 33: 89–91
72. Van Ketel WG, Bruynzeel DP, Bezemer PD, Stamhuis HI (1984) Toxicity of handcleaners. Dermatologica 168: 94–99
73. Werner Y, Lindberg (1985) Transepidermal water loss in dry and clinically normal skin in patients with atopic dermatitis. Acta Derm Venereol (Stockh) 65: 102–105

*Quality Assurance
and Environmental Aspects
of Synthetic Detergent Skin Cleansers*

Biopharmaceutical Aspects of Synthetic Detergent Skin Cleansers

K. Thoma

Introduction

Biopharmacy is an interdisciplinary science that looks at the way in which pharmaceutical technology (the formulation of active and ancillary substances into actual products) interacts with the processes in the living organism.

At first sight, it might appear that, to the pharmaceutical technologist engaged in the development of drug formulations, synthetic detergent skin cleansers are of only marginal importance.

However, while synthetic cleansers are much used for cosmetic skin care, and are covered by the Cosmetics Regulations, they are also of considerable importance in the treatment of skin disorders.

In looking at the biopharmaceutical aspects – how to achieve the desirable effects and how to prevent the unwanted ones – from the point of view of product quality, we shall, inevitably, be going over some of the ground covered in previous papers at this Symposium.

Advantages and Efficacy of Skin Cleansers

Figure 1 shows the potential benefits of synthetic detergent skin cleansers, which have to be translated into product formulations and assured by quality control.

One undoubted advantage of synthetic detergents is their pH adjustability which makes it possible to adapt the product to the physiological pH level, or to choose a different level for therapeutical purposes.

If it is decided to adjust the product to an acidic pH, e.g. by the addition of citric acid, attention should be paid, not only to the target pH, but also to the buffering capacity of the system.

Others have already dealt with the fact that, by comparison with alkaline soaps, these pH adjusted synthetic cleansers cause only minor changes in skin pH.

As will be seen from Fig. 2, the skin pH of unwashed skin (A) of 6.0 to 6.5 is raised to above pH 9.0 by washing with alkaline soap [10].

One hour after washing, the pH of the dry skin is between 6.8 and 7.5, which means that it has not fully recovered by that time.

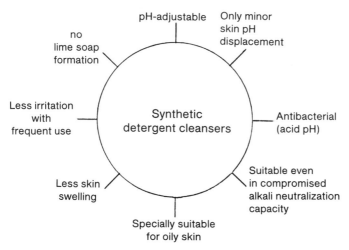

Fig. 1. Actions and benefits of synthetic detergent skin cleansers

The same study (Fig. 3) showed a similar response when a synthetic cleanser (II) containing alkaline soap was used. Alkali-free washing is guaranteed only by synthetic cleansers 3A and III.

Weakly acid synthetic cleansers can be beneficial in the adjuvant treatment of skin disorders. Antimycotic and antibacterial effects in intertriginous areas have been confirmed by experimental studies, as shown in Fig. 4 [4].

For Corynebacterium acnes, this inhibition was found even at dilutions of 1:1000 under anaerobic conditions. These findings, as well as others, suggest that certain synthetic detergents are bacteriostatic. However, it will be seen from the example given that aqueous detergent solutions cannot be expected to cover the entire microbial spectrum, neither can they completely prevent colonization.

Figure 1 shows three further dermatologically useful features of synthetic detergent preparations: These agents can be used even if the skin's alkali neutralization capacity is diminished; they are particularly suitable for seborrhoeic skins; and their alkali-free composition produces much less skin swelling, thereby preventing the occlusion of the sweat and sebaceous glands seen in the swollen stratum corneum following the use of alkaline soaps [1].

Alkaline soaps produce lime soaps, which are deposited on the skin and can exacerbate dermatitic lesions; hence the dermatologists' advice that dermatitis patients should avoid soap. Synthetic detergents do not form lime soaps, and therefore do not suffer from the same restrictions of use.

Also, synthetic detergents are not hard water sensitive. As a result, they have the major advantage in everyday use of not causing bathtub ring or scum.

Mildness is a particularly important feature of a product intended for frequent use [8].

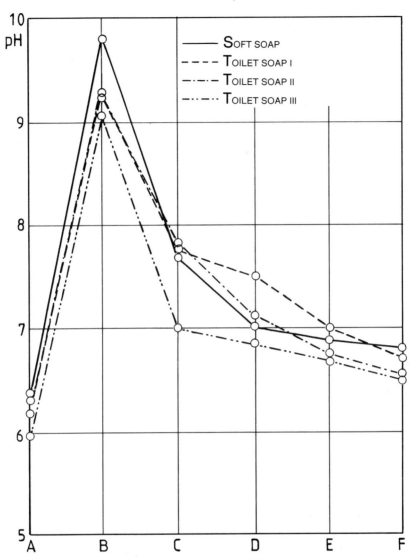

Fig. 2. Skin pH before, during, and after washing with different soaps, under actual use conditions (water hardnness 20° German hardness; water temperature 20°C. A = unwashed skin; B = lathered skin; C = washed, well rinsed skin; D = dry skin, 1 hour after washing [10]

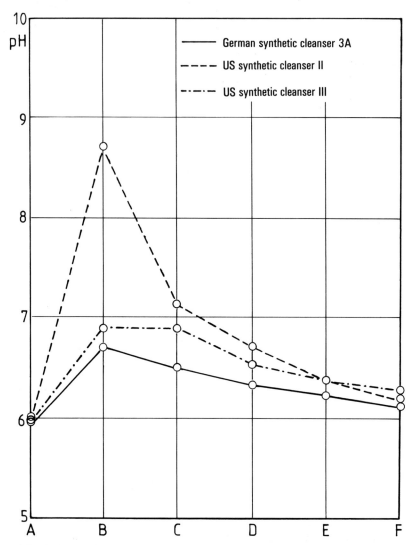

Fig. 3. Skin before, during, and after washing with different synthetic detergent cleansers under actual use conditions (water hardness 20° German hardness; water temperature 20 °C) [10]

However, since even the mildest product may be irritating if wrongly used, information must be provided to tell the consumer how to use the product (water temperature, concentration, frequency and duration of use).

In principle, all of the beneficial features discussed above can be incorporated in a synthetic cleanser that will cater for people with sensitive skins and those who work in occupations that require them to wash frequently. For optimum product design, several essential requirements will have to be taken into account.

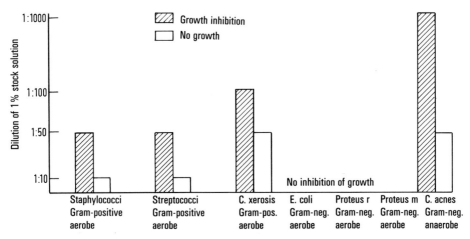

Fig. 4. Investigation of inhibition by seba med of bacterial growth [4]

It is obvious that frequent thorough cleansing can be a source of skin irritation, brought about by the removal in the washing liquor of the water soluble constituents of the natural moisturizing factor (NMF), protein denaturation by surfactants, and, especially, by the continual removal of natural skin lipids [9].

As the water binding capacity of the stratum corneum is decreased, water will be lost, and the skin will become dry and rough.

Product Quality and Ingredients

For a cleanser to be good or, indeed, better than others, it must provide the required cleansing action while causing as little irritation as possible, even when used repeatedly [6].

On the raw material (surfactant) side, care must be taken to choose substances of suitable ionic nature, structure, and chain length (Fig. 5). Whereas, among the anionic surfactants, the C12 compound sodium lauryl sulphate has considerable irritancy, milder products can be formulated using less irritant anionic surfactants such as the sulphosuccinates or ethoxylated alkyl sulphates [5].

Nonionic surfactants such as fatty alcohol polyglycol ethers or polysorbates are milder yet, while protein fatty acid condensates and amphoteric surfactants are particularly well tolerated [7, 5].

As will be seen from Table 1, the excess skin water loss caused by a sodium lauryl sulphate solution can be markedly decreased, and the increase in roughness after drying mitigated, when Tego-betaine L7, an amphoteric surfactant, is added to the mixture [9].

Anionic surfactants
   Na-lauryl sulphate
   Na-lauryl ether sulphate
   Na-sulphosuccinate

Nonionic surfactants
   Fatty alcohol polyglycol ethers

Amphoteric surfactants
   Cocoamidopropyl betaines

Protein fatty acid condensation products

Fig. 5. Surfactant categories in ascending order of skin compatibility

Figure 6 shows that the addition of 20% protein fatty acid condensate will give an improvement by about 60% in the mucous membrane compatibility of the anionic surfactant [7].

In the formulation of a suitably mild synthetic detergent product, attention must be paid to the fatty agents. These substances are added in order to restore the lipids removed by washing.

Different classes of chemicals are available to suit different purposes. Thus there are

- spreadability enhancing agents, such as isopropyl myristate or palmitate;
- hydrophilized lipids, such as ethoxylated fatty alcohols, or
- mono- or diglycerides of fatty acids, such as lauric acid monoglyceride [2, 3].

It is true that such protective lipids added for emolliency may somewhat diminish the detergency of the cleansers; however, they are of major importance for product tolerability (Fig. 7).

Table 1. Effects of ampholyte additions on the action of sodium lauryl sulphate [9]

Surfactant	Detergency	Alkali neutralization	Skin water loss	Change in resonance frequency	Skin roughness
Sodium lauryl sulphate (2% solution)	72.4%	511	83.6%	−1	+7.4
Mixture (1:1) of SLS/TEGO betaine L7	68.5%	455	67.8%	+1	+2.8
TEGO betaine L7 (2% solution)	61.6%	464	71.4%	−1	+0.9
Control	–	416	–	–	–

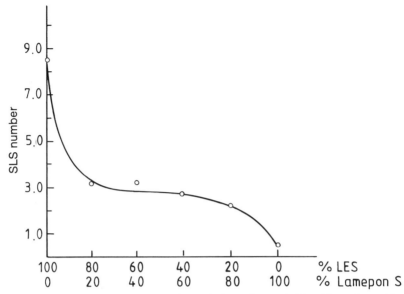

Fig. 6. Rabbit eye irritancy of a combination of lauryl ether sulphate (LES) with a polypeptide fatty acid condensate (Lamepon S) in a 2% solution [7]

Tables 2 and 3 show the factors that should be taken into account in the formulation of the two types of synthetic detergent cleansers.

While alkaline soap is not, in principle, an ingredient of the formula, it may be added to the mixture of anionic and amphoteric surfactants. The solids – kaolin or paraffin – are added to give body to the bar-type cleansers. pH adjustment is by means of organic acids, such as lactic acid or citric acid. The example in Table 2 shows that antioxidants and chelating agents may be added to achieve chemical stabilization of unsaturated constituents. The formulation given does not list the residual water content, which may be between 3 and 10%.

Unlike most of the liquid cleansers, synthetic cleanser bars do not require the addition of preservatives.

Cleanser bars are subject to "sloughing" – going soft and sludging – in water, and therefore have to be kept on a dry surface.

The liquid cleanser formulation shows a water content of between 60 and 80%. In this case, the surfactant content is about 15–20%; foam stabilizers and thickeners may be added to improve product performance. The formula given has been superfatted with lanolin oil, while the pH has been adjusted using citric acid.

Since the water content is comparatively high, a preservative is usually required.

The second edition of Unwanted Effects of Cosmetics And Drugs Used in Dermatology (1985) lists no data on side effects of liquid cleansers [5]. This is

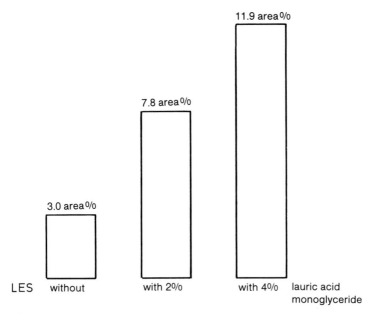

Fig. 7. Lipid restoration by 2% and 4% lauric acid monoglyceride in 20% sodium lauryl ether sulphate solutions used for forearm immersion [2] (lauric acid monoglyceride in % of skin lipids extracted from a 20 cm² surface area)

Table 2. Typical formula of a syndet soap bar (after Nater and de Groot [5])

Ingredients		Example
50–95%	synthetic surfactant	dioctyl sodium sulphosuccinate, sodium lauryl sulphate, cocoamidopropyl betaine
0–50%	soap: sodium salt of fatty acids	sodium cocoate
5–20%	additives to aid technological performance	kaolin, sorbitol, paraffin, sodium silicate, cellulose gum
1–5%	pH adjusting agent (to a pH of ca. 5.5)	lactic acid, citric acid
ca. 0.1%	antioxidant and chelating agent	Sopant, edetic acid
ca. 0.5%	perfume	perfume

in line with the general observation that allergic reactions to synthetic detergent cleansers are rare occurrences.

As far as preservatives are concerned, the risk of time-dependent side effects may be taken to be non-existent, since the skin contact time is short and the cleanser is removed by rinsing.

Table 3. Typical formula for a handwashing lotion (handcleaner) (after Nater and de Groot [5])

Ingredients		Example[a]
60–80%	water	water
ca. 15%	surfactant	Amphoteric-2, disodium monoundecylen-amido-monoethanolamine sulphosuccinate
ca. 1%	surfactant: foam builder	lauramide monoethanolamide
ca. 1%	thickener	Carbomer-934
ca. 2%	lipid: superfatting agent	lanolin oil
ca. 1%	organic acid: pH adjusting agent	citric acid
ca. 0.3%	preservative	Kathon CG[b]
ca. 0.01%	colour	C.I. 19140
ca. 0.3%	perfume	perfume

[a] Foreign products intended for sale in the Federal Republic of Germany must comply with the FRG Cosmetics Regulation. Products that do not meet the requirements will be banned, even if they are permitted in other countries.
[b] The above example gives Kathon CG as a preservative. This mixture of two isothiazolones is causing concern about possible side effects. Therefore, under the Cosmetics Regulation, the maximum permitted concentration is now only 0.0015%.

The design of an optimal synthetic cleanser product that will be widely used while causing minimal irritation even in sensitive skins and with frequent use is a complex matter. All aspects of the formulation – pH, buffering capacity, surfactant combinations and concentrations, raw materials and ancillary substances – have to be carefully matched and balanced in order to come up with a product that is safe and acceptable.

References

1. Braun-Falco O, Heilgemeir GP (1981) Syndets zur Reinigung gesunder und erkrankter Haut. Ther Gegenw 120: 1028
2. Domsch AW (1986) Rückfettung in Bade- und Duschpräparaten. Seifen–Öle–Fette–Wachse 112: 163
3. Gloor M, Voss H-J, Kionke M, Friedrich HC (1972) Entfettung und Rückfettung der Haut bei Körperreinigung durch tensidhaltige Lösungen mit Lipidzusätzen. Therapiewoche 22: 4236

4. Marghescu S (1970) Die Intertrigo, ihre Prophylaxe und Behandlung. Ther Gegenw 109: 813
5. Nater JP, de Groot AC (1985) Unwanted Effects of Cosmetics and Drugs used in Dermatology. 2nd Edition, Elsevier, Amsterdam New York Oxford, p 348
6. Proksch E (1987) Anforderungen des Dermatologen an Badepräparate. Seifen – Öle – Fette – Wachse 113: 79
7. Schuster G, Modde H, Scheld E (1965) Eiweißfettsäurekondensate – ihre Eigenschaften und Anwendung. Seifen – Öle – Fette – Wachse 91: 477
8. Siemer E, Elmahdi K (1987) Empfindliche Haut: Probleme – Pflege – Beratung. Pharm Ztg 132: 2135
9. Tronnier H (1981) Irritative Waschmittelschädigungen. Experiment und Klinik. Parfümerie und Kosmetik 62: 388
10. Werdelmann B (1958) Untersuchungen zur Hautwirksamkeit moderner Körperreinigungsmittel: Pufferkapazität und Hautreaktion. Berufsdermatosen 6: 250

Quality Control of Synthetic Detergent Cleansers

K. Stanzl

Introduction

This paper deals with the quality control of surfactants to be used in synthetic cleansers, using the example of sodium cocoyl isethionate. Problems involved will be described, and solutions proposed.

Influence of the Manufacturing Process on Product Quality

The raw materials used in the manufacture of cleanser bars come in three categories:
a) Surfactants,
b) Emollients/moisturizers,
c) Fillers.

Let us assume that sodium cocoyl isethionate has been chosen as the surfactant constituent, because of its mildness, hard water tolerance, and good lathering. Once this decision has been taken, the Quality Assurance department will start looking into the manufacturing process implications.

The esters of isethionic acid

$R - COOC_2H_4SO_3Na$

are obtained from coconut oleic or myristic acids [1].

There are various methods by which these esters may be produced:

All methods start from isethionic acid, which is obtained from ethylene and sulphur trioxide (Fig. 1) [2].

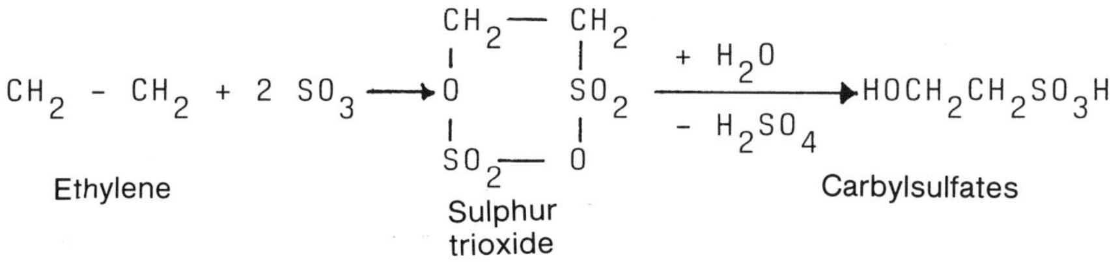

$$CH_2 - CH_2 + 2\,SO_3 \longrightarrow \begin{array}{c} CH_2 - CH_2 \\ | \quad\quad | \\ O \quad\quad SO_2 \\ | \quad\quad | \\ SO_2 - O \end{array} \xrightarrow[-\,H_2SO_4]{+\,H_2O} HOCH_2CH_2SO_3H$$

Ethylene   Sulphur trioxide   Carbylsulfates

Fig. 1. Production of isethionic acid

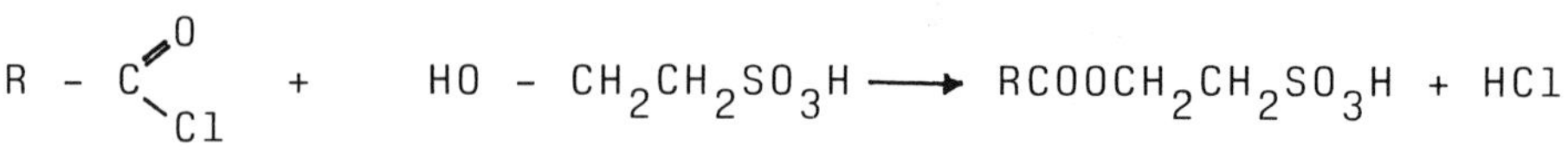

$$R - C\overset{\displaystyle O}{\underset{\displaystyle Cl}{\diagdown}} \quad + \quad HO - CH_2CH_2SO_3H \longrightarrow RCOOCH_2CH_2SO_3H + HCl$$

R = fatty acid ester

Fig. 2a. Production of sodium cocyl isethionate from fatty acid chloride

In one of the methods, isethionic acid is reacted with fatty acid chlorides (Fig. 2a) obtained from the interaction of the fatty acid with PCl₃ (Fig. 2b).

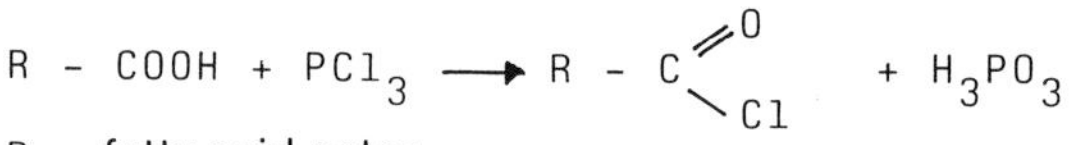

$$R - COOH + PCl_3 \longrightarrow R - C\overset{\displaystyle O}{\underset{\displaystyle Cl}{\diagdown}} + H_3PO_3$$

R = fatty acid ester

Fig. 2b. Production of fatty acid chloride

The final product contains a number of impurities. Apart from organophosphorus compounds, there will be free fatty acids or inorganic salts of isethionic acid in the raw material.

It is also possible to use the direct esterification of the fatty acid with the sodium salt of isethionic acid (Fig. 2c).

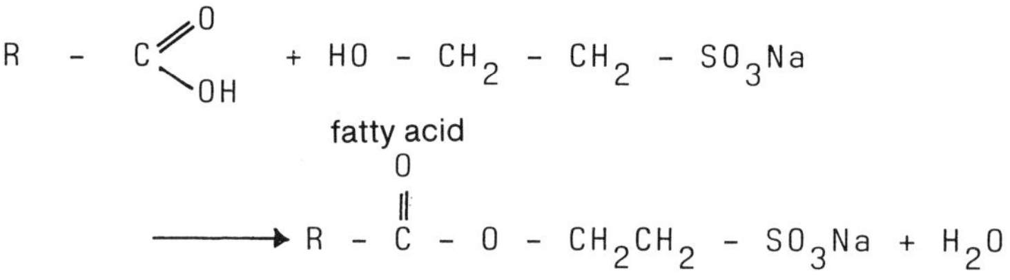

$$R - C\overset{\displaystyle O}{\underset{\displaystyle OH}{\diagdown}} + HO - CH_2 - CH_2 - SO_3Na$$

fatty acid

$$\longrightarrow R - \overset{\overset{\displaystyle O}{\|}}{C} - O - CH_2CH_2 - SO_3Na + H_2O$$

Fig. 2c. Production of sodium cocoyl isethionate by direct esterification

There is a principal difference between the two methods: In the former (acid chloride) method, common salt is produced as an electrolyte; this is not the case with the direct esterification method.

However, even if the same method for the production of sodium cocoyl isethionate is employed, different reaction conditions may result in different levels of byproducts in the isethionates produced.

The table below lists two typical analyses of sodium cocoyl isethionate:

	A	B
Na-cocoyl isethionate	75 %	85.6 %
Free fatty acid	19 %	3.5 %
NaCl	0 %	0 %
Na-isethionate	0.5 %	6.8 %

It should be obvious that the different proportions of byproducts will affect the properties of the end product. The physico-chemical properties, such as stability, pH, or viscosity, will vary, as will skin compatibility.

Therefore, the influence of each byproduct on the product properties will have to be studied. After that the detailed raw material specification has to be drawn up. If, for instance, it is found that the amount of free sodium isethionate will affect the wear of a cleanser bar, the specification will have to lay down limits for this constituent. Equally, there must be limits specified for the proportion of sodium cocoyl isethionate. A look at the table given above will show that in case A, the customer would be getting only 75% of actual surfactant for his money, whereas in case B, the amount would be 85.6%.

One important criterion for user acceptance is sloughing, i.e. the ability of the cleanser bar to absorb water, with more absorption producing greater softening of the bar.

Sloughing is determined under very realistic conditions, by hanging the bar in water for a certain period of time, then drying it, and removing the softened outer layer.

The amount of sloughing is very much a function of the formula chosen. However, other factors enter into the process as well, as was seen when bars made to the same formula by two different manufacturers were found to produce different sloughing values.

Quality Assurance must work together with Research and Development to find the optimum manufacturing process that will give consistent product quality.

Important Product Quality Criteria

One way of finding out what the user requires in terms of quality is a survey among the target group. The chief problem, no doubt, is the definition of this group, and the correct selection of a representative sample. It may be assumed that the most important features of cleanser bars, from the point of view of the user, are cleansing power, mildness, fragrance, and long life.

Cleansing power should not, normally, be a problem, since the surfactant content of the product will be high.

Mildness may be a problem, for the same reason. Surfactants can cause roughness, swelling, and irritation of the skin, as well as changing skin permeability and hydration.

All these aspects must be considered during development, since, later on, no amount of quality control will alter the properties of the product.

Fragrance should be preserved for several years, provided that the product has been carefully formulated and manufactured.

Economy in use (the *dish life* of the product) – a major consideration to the price-conscious user – is mainly a function of
– the composition,
– the manufacture,

– the age, and
– the type of storage of the cleanser bar.

The faster a bar is allowed to dissolve, the less long-lived it will be. This is why it is important not to keep cleanser bars in a pool of water.

Modern cleanser formulations strike a balance between the ready solubility required for quick lathering, and the slower solubility that makes for long product life.

Since cleanser bars contain high concentrations of surfactants and very little water, they do not provide a hospitable environment for micro-organisms.

The situation is different with liquid cleansers. These cleansers are a major challenge to the formulator, since they have to be both biodegradable and biologically stable while in use. In other words, it should be possible for micro-organisms in the sewage treatment plant to break them down; but micro-organisms are not allowed to cause spoilage during normal use.

Several biodegradable surfactants may have a pH and an osmolality that make them stable; however, this stability is concentration-dependent, and will be affected once the agent is diluted. Figure 3 shows just how concentration sensitive surfactants are [3].

In the first case, all the micro-organisms introduced are killed within three days. However, if the concentration of the surfactant is reduced to 20% and below, it will be seen – especially with Pseudomonas aeruginosa – that the original count fails to decrease; and once the concentration drops below 10%, the same pattern is seen for all the test organisms used.

Micro-organisms are a form of "growing contamination" [4]. The problem comes, not only from the living organisms, but from the enzymes formed by them. Most of the time, the enzymes will remain active even if the enzyme-producing bacteria and fungi have been killed by chemical preservatives. It is, therefore, vital for the manufacturer to observe scrupulous hygiene throughout the manufacturing process, in order to keep out micro-organisms and to ensure that the product will reach the user in perfect condition and retain microbiological purity while it is in the user's possession.

For this requirement to be met, antimicrobial preservatives will have to be added to the product. The selection of the preservative to be used in a particular cleanser will depend on the nature of the product, as well as on the dermatological and toxicological profile of the agent itself.

Micro-organisms – "bugs" – are everywhere, on the skin, in the air, in water. It is from these media that they are transferred into the product.

Spoilage is not necessarily the work of pathogens, but can equally be brought about by (non-pathogenic) environmental micro-organisms.

In summary, Quality is not something that is put into a product by controls, however carefully done: It is an ingredient that has to be designed into the product from the word go.

Quality Control of Synthetic Detergent Cleansers 207

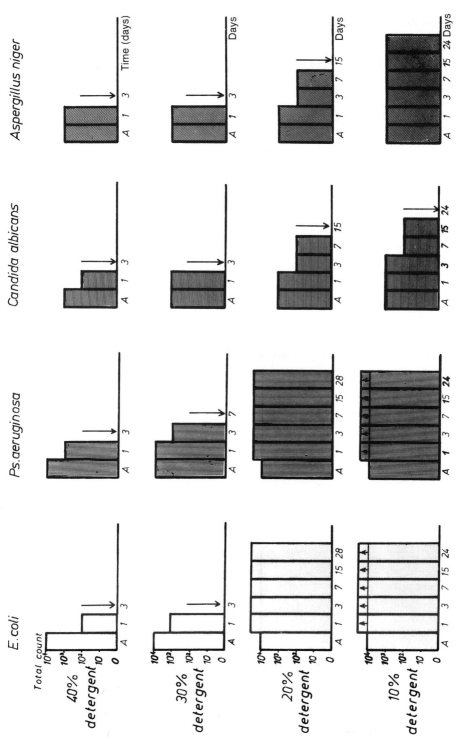

Fig. 3. Surfactant susceptibility to micro-organisms as a function of concentrations (from [3])

References

1. GAF Igepon Anionic Surfactant Bulletin, Frechen 1971
2. Longman GF The Analysis of Detergents and Detergent Products, John Wiley & Sons, Chichester New York Brisbane Toronto
3. Wallhäußer KH (1974) Die Konservierung von Waschmitteln und Kosmetika. Seifen, Öle, Fette, Wachse 100: 571–574, 577–588
4. Rieger M (1985) Surfactants in Cosmetics. Marcel Dekker, New York, p 219

Environmental Aspects of Synthetic Detergent Preparations

H. H. Rump

Background

With the increased use of synthetic detergent preparations for body care, the question of the way in which these substances affect the environment (especially water) is becoming more and more important. Although the amounts of synthetic detergents contributed to the effluent and, hence, to the environmental burden, by body care products are small compared with the quantities produced by other detergent uses, they must not be overlooked.

The surfactants contained in synthetic detergent products reduce the surface tension of water, to permit wetting of the skin and the removal of soil particles. The environmentalists' concern is, firstly, with the possible adverse effects of detergents on the aquatic biological community (organisms such as bacteria, daphnia, algae, and fish), and, secondly, with the biodegradability of the compounds involved. From the environmental point of view, it would be preferable for substances to have low toxicity to aquatic organisms, and to be readily degradable in sewage treatment plants, lakes and rivers.

There is no immediate correlation between the toxicity and the degradability of a substance or a product. The persistence of a compound does not permit conclusions to be drawn as to its toxicity; and toxicity data cannot be used to assess the degradability of a substance. There are three aspects of biodegradation:

1. Primary biodegradation, which is usually complete once an essential functional group has been lost, changing the chemical identity of the substance.
2. Environmentally acceptable degradation, which means the removal of nuisance properties (e.g. detergent foaming).
3. Ultimate biodegradability, i.e. the complete mineralization of the organic constituents of a substance, which results in a harmless end product.

The frequently used term "elimination" refers to the removal of a substance from the water, though not from the environment as a whole. Thus, elimination can be brought about by adsorption to solids, a physical process that does not involve any chemical transformation or mineralization. This should be borne in mind when listening to claims that a particular substance is "environment friendly" or "compatible with the environment."

Synthetic Detergent Cleansers and the Aquatic Environment

Tests to assess the behaviour of substances in the environment suffer from several problems. Firstly, the simulation of the natural conditions in sewage treatment plants, rivers, etc., must be sufficiently realistic to permit predictions to be made. Secondly, the tests must be reproducible, a requirement that is not easy to meet in biological testing.

Influence on Aquatic Organisms

The effect on aquatic organisms is governed by various factors:
- pH
- incubation temperature
- concentration of the substance
- amount of substrate
- nature of the substrate
- duration of exposure
- adsorption characteristics of the substance
- type of organisms.

While pH, incubation temperature, substance concentration, and amount of substrate can be agreed for environmental tests, the nature of the substrate is less straightforward. If it is decided to use only effluent or admixtures of effluent, (since, after all, the object of the test is to determine the effect of the substance on the mixed bacterial species in sewage), the results may vary widely depending on the source of the effluent. Using a defined substrate such as glucose or peptone will not solve the problem, since the pattern of living organisms in such a substrate may be fundamentally different from that in real sewage.

The duration of exposure is another important quantity in the determination of toxicity. The inhibitory effect is given by the equation

$$H = k \cdot cdt$$

where the inhibitory effect I is an integral of the substance concentration c over the measuring time t, and where specific characteristics are represented by the factor k.

Adsorption and the inoculate used can have a major influence on the toxicity of substances. The use of large amounts of activated sludge as an inoculum may not correctly reflect toxicity.

Figure 1 shows that, with the use of mixed bacterial species, the toxic effect declines, after some time, to a very low value, as a function of the adsorption isotherm of the test substance. This means that most of the test substance will have become fixed, and will, therefore, no longer be toxic to freely moving micro-organisms.

In toxicity testing, one frequently used parameter is the change in the gas metabolism of micro-organisms. These studies involve the measurement, in

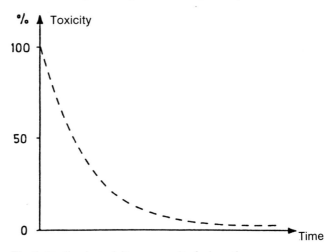

Fig. 1. Decline in toxicity as a result of adsorption

closed systems and over an extended period (5 days), of the oxygen uptake rate of the micro-organisms, using small volumes of effluent or peptone as the inoculum. The same method is customarily used for the direct determination of the biochemical oxygen demand (BOD).

Whereas ordinary BOD assays will almost exclusively measure substrate metabolism, respirometric techniques also include the endogenous respiration of bacteria and protozoan respiration.

The presence of toxic or inhibitory substances will decrease the oxygen demand of the micro-organisms. The decrease in the oxygen demand provides a measure of the degree of inhibition. Test runs are done with substance-and-substrate samples, and with blank (substrate-only) controls. At the end of the test, the data from the three samples used are plotted as graphs. The area under the BOD curve is proportional to the oxygen consumption. The area obtained with a substance-and -substrate sample is then compared with the area under the curve resulting from substrate only, to see whether there has been inhibition of respiration. Figure 2 shows the application of this technique to a body care product. The lowest curve shows respiration in the sample containing the synthetic detergent cleanser; the curve above represents respiration in the readily degraded substrate (peptone), while the topmost curve was obtained using a mixture of substance and peptone.

The illustration contains a fourth, broken line, which represents the calculated summation curve of the two upper graphs. If peptone degradation had been inhibited by the synthetic detergent, the broken line would be uppermost. Since that is not the case in Figure 2, it may be concluded that the detergent does not inhibit degradation. Indeed, degradation is more rapid. If inhibition is found, the area between the expected and the actually measured curves is integrated ("inhibition area"), and specified in per cent to quantify the toxicity of the test substance.

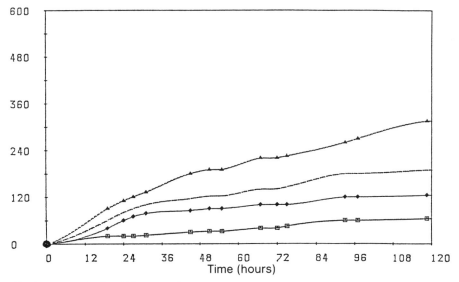

Fig. 2. Respiration inhibition test of a synthetic detergent cleanser

Biodegradability

Problems Inherent in the Different Test Methods

Sections 1 and 3 of the German Detergents Act stipulate that all surfactants used in laundry detergents must be sufficiently biodegradable and eliminable in sewage treatment plants. While this requirement is not explicitly made for synthetic cleansers, it would be desirable for these products to be equally biodegradable.

Primary biodegradability, as mentioned above, gives a measure of the degree to which surfactant molecules lose their surface active properties; without, however, indicating what happens to the fragments of molecules that remain once primary degradation is complete.

There is a range of OECD tests for the biodegradability of products, including
- ready biodegradability tests,
- inherent biodegradability tests, and
- simulation tests.

The choice of test – from the long list of possible techniques – will be a function of the specific problem to be studied. One frequently used method employs a simulation of sewage treatment plants. The OECD confirmatory test used for this purpose permits the study, by means of special analytical techniques, of the primary degradability of, for instance, anionic surfactants. However, the technique cannot be applied to the testing of complex product formulations. In such cases, static tests have proved useful, employing DOC (dissolved organic carbon) or COD (chemical oxygen demand) as parameters. Reference [1] gives information on where these tests can be used, as well as details of the methodologies.

Degradation of Surfactants and Finished Detergent Products

Measurements of the degradability of individual substances or groups of substances may be difficult because, in order to be studied, the substances have to be removed from their substrate. In straightforward cases, foam stripping can be done, followed by Fourier Transform IR spectrometry to identify the surfactant mixture isolated [2]. Curve 1 in Figure 3 shows an unknown mixture with strong IR absorption bands at 2800, 2400, 1700, and 1100 cm^{-1}. The computer will compare the spectrum in Curve 1 with library spectra, and suggest a substance. The product shown obviously contained an alkylol amide (Curve 2). After the subtraction of the alkylol amide spectrum from the spectrum of the mixture, the spectrum in Figure 4 was obtained. The substance was identified as a fatty acid polyglycol ether.

The changes in the patterns of the various constituents of a synthetic cleanser when tested for degradability using OECD Test 302 B can be shown with pyrolysis field ionization mass spectrometry (PFIMS), using soft ionization methods. The technique is described in [3]. The following changes are observed:

The original product contains ions, e.g. at m/z 517, 561, 605, 649, 693, 737, 781, and 825. The differences of 44 mass units each would suggest the presence in the mixture of ethylene oxide ($CH_2CH_2O^-$) units (Fig. 5).

In the sample examined after 21 days of degradation testing, the masses found in the initial product between m/z 517 and m/z 825 have disappeared, i.e. these substances have been completely degraded (Fig. 6).

Reference [4] gives details of the intermediate steps by which degradation can proceed.

Figure 7 shows an empirical example of the degradation of a synthetic cleanser in OECD Test 302 B. It will be seen that within a short time there is much elimination of DOC, some of which may be due to adsorption to solid surfaces. This initial elimination phase is followed by a gradual decrease in the amounts of product constituents, ultimately reaching an excellent degradation (elimination) level of 97%.

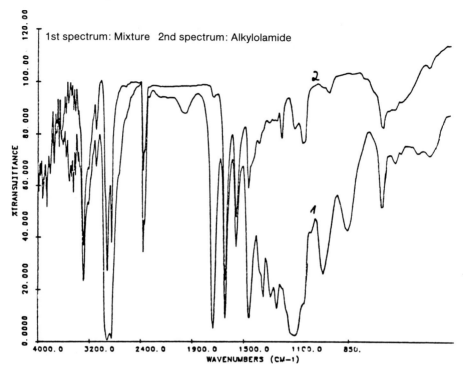

Fig. 3. FT-IR spectra of a surfactant mixture and of a single constituent

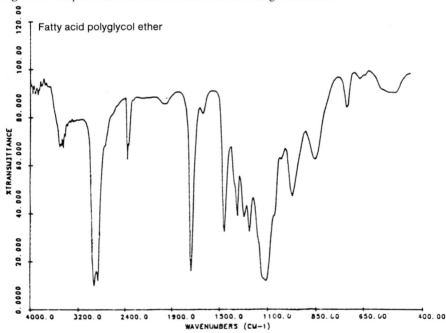

Fig. 4. FT-IR spectrum of a synthetic cleanser ingredient

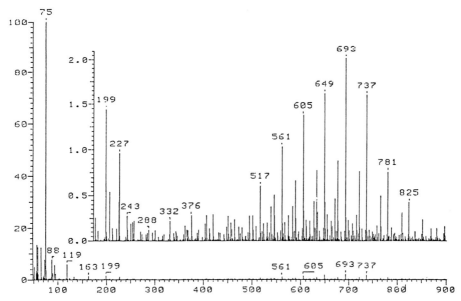

Fig. 5. PFIMS spectrum of a synthetic cleanser formulation before degradation

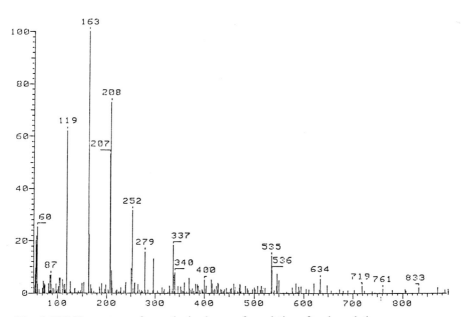

Fig. 6. PFIMS spectrum of a synthetic cleanser formulation after degradation

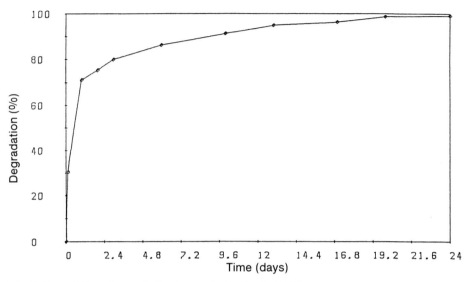

Fig. 7. Degradation of a synthetic cleanser in OECD Test 302 B

References

1. OECD (ed) (1981) OECD-guidelines for the testing of chemicals. Paris
2. Rump HH, Fischer G, Gilles T (1985) Anwendungsmöglichkeiten der rechnerunterstützten Fourier-Transformations-IR-Spektrometrie. Gewässerschutz – Wasser – Abwasser 79: 338–351
3. Schulten HR, Halket JM (1986) Rapid characterisation of biomaterials. Org Mass Spectrom 21: 613
4. Swisher RD (1987) Surfactant biodegradation 2nd ed, New York

The Use of Synthetic Detergent Skin Cleansers

The Use of Synthetic Detergent Skin Cleansers – The Cosmetic Chemists's View

H. P. Fiedler

Background

Throughout his existence as a social being, Man has tried to impress and attract others in the community by looking good – even enhancing the natural appearance by the use of ornamental colour – and smelling nice. In fact, what we now call cosmetics has been a human concern from the most primitive times.

Of course, improving one's appearance – beautification – is not the only purpose for which cosmetics are used. The broadest definition of cosmetics includes also toiletries – items used for personal grooming, to keep the body sweet and clean. Indeed, there would even appear to be a higher, spiritual dimension to the use of such agents. It is said that cleanliness is next to godliness – something the ancient Egyptians learned from their priests, who would not allow the faithful to enter the temple until they had bathed and anointed themselves. Significantly, the first records of the manufacture and use of soap come from that part of the world. Some 4500 years ago, the Sumerians, a Semitic people, were using fat and wood ashes to obtain a substance that made the washing of clothes easier and which, apparently, was also successful as a skin cleanser [9].

In the 2nd century A. D., the Greek physician Galen, who practised in Rome, described a product made from fat and wood ashes which he called sapo and to which he attributed not only cleansing but also wound-healing properties.

The decline of the Roman Empire was followed by the soapless centuries, when washing and bathing (especially the use of public baths) were frowned upon or actually banned. This time of low standards of personal care was followed by an age in which soap was once again becoming increasingly important. It is interesting to note that the soaps then used were of the same chemical pattern as their modern counterparts (alkali salts of higher fatty acids). Also, as soap was becoming an item of daily use rather than a luxury, there was increasing awareness of the need for skin and hair cleansing, in order to keep these structures healthy as well as making them more attractive [8].

After A. Marchionini et al. had shown that the moisture layer covering the skin gives a mainly acid reaction, which is of critical importance for the resistance of the skin to microbial attack, other researchers soon found that soap solutions – with their inherently alkaline pH – were not best suited for skin cleansing, and that even water – as a hypotonic agent – was far from ideal.

In spite of these findings, soap has remained the primary skin cleanser to this day, probably because of its ease of handling and storage, and also because the quality and skin compatibility of soaps have been greatly improved [1].

Synthetic Surfactants

Despite the universal use of soap, attempts had been made all along to find other substances with similar properties. Various naturally occurring agents had been tried and found more or less wanting, when, in a different field of research, sulphonates were found to be superior to soap as laundering agents. This discovery ushered in the development of synthetic surfactants and detergents.

The first successful work was done by two German chemists, H. Bertsch and G. Schuster, working at Boehme Fettchemie GmbH. In 1928, these scientists found a way of obtaining fatty acids from fats; fatty alcohols from the fatty acids; and, finally, fatty alcohol sulphates from the alcohols.

The substances thus produced were water soluble, giving clear, neutral, colourless and odourless solutions of excellent detergency. These fatty alcohol sulphates were used early on (1932) for FEWA, the first light-duty detergent to be marketed.

There were, of course, immediate attempts to see whether these new substances could be used, not only as laundry agents, but also for skin cleansing, e.g. by making them into a solid cleanser bar. However, despite the neutral reaction of the synthetic detergent solutions, the products were totally unsuitable for skin care. The benefits of excellent detergency were cancelled out by excessive defatting and drying of the skin, with removal of substances from the horny layer which were later found to be vital for skin hydration.

Disappointing though they were, these initial findings served to stimulate research in university hospitals and in industry, prompting more co-operation between dermatologists and cosmetic chemists.

It is obviously impossible to go into all the details of the further history; a mention of some of the milestones will have to suffice.

Surfactants for Skin Cleansing

The list of surfactants reported to be suitable also for skin cleansing became longer and longer, and has been growing to this day, when there are many monographs – some of them in several volumes – on these agents [7]. Next, the suggestion was made to use the terms "tensides" to cover all surfactants (including, of course, soap) [4], and to describe the properties of these tensides in a draft German DIN standard. The standard produced as a result of this work was DIN 59900, listing tensides (surfactants) as anionic, ampholytic, cationic, or nonionic.

Dermatologists, industrial chemists, and cosmetic chemists were closely working together to select surfactants with particular suitability as gentle skin cleansers. Lists of these agents can be found in the literature [2, 3]. One such list of candidate surfactants for skin cleansers is given below.

Anionic surfactants

Soaps
Alkyl ether sulphates
Alkyl sulphates
Sulphosuccinic acid mono- and diesters
Sec. alkane sulphonates, hydroxy alkane sulphonates, a-olefin sulphonates and a-sulpho fatty acid methyl esters
Alkyl amide ether sulphates
Fatty acid condensation products
Protein fatty acid condensation products
Fatty acid sarcosinates
Fatty acid methyl taurates
Fatty acid isethionates
Alkyl ether phosphates
Monoglyceride sulphates

Cationic Surfactants

Cetyl trimethyl ammonium bromide and chloride
Distearyl dimethyl ammonium chloride
Benzyl dimethyl stearyl ammonium chloride

Amphoteric Surfactants

Alkyl betaines
Alkyl imidazolinium betaines
Alkyl sulpho betaines
Amidoalkyl betaines
N-alkyl-ß-amino propionates
N-alkyl-ß-imino propionates

Nonionic Surfactants

Fatty alcohol polyglycol ethers
Alkylphenol polyglycol ethers
(octylphenol or nonylphenol polyethyleneglycol ethers)
Fatty acid polyglycol esters
(stearic acid esters)
Ethylene oxide-propylene oxide block polymers
Ethoxylated fatty acid monoglyderides

Polyglycerine fatty acid esters
Sugar esters
(saccharose palmitate)
Pentaerythritol partial esters
Ethoxylated pentaerythritol partial esters
Sorbitan fatty acid esters
Ethoxylated sorbitan fatty acid esters
Fatty acid alkanol amides and dialkanol amides
Fatty acid alkanol amide polyglycol ethers
Fatty amine oxides
Fatty acid monoglycerides
Fatty acid glycol partial esters
(diethylene glycol monostereate)

Not all the available surfactants are equally suitable for the formulation of gentle skin cleansers. The cosmetic chemist will have to use his experience and his knowledge to put together certain surfactants of specific and/or known properties in an optimum product formula. Other substances, such as superfatting agents, skin protectants or anti-irritants [5], etc., may be added to the surfactant mixture. Technical experience, testing facilities, and the input from the dermatologists can be used to formulate a skin cleanser that will live up to the expectations of the dermatologists and of the actual users.

The technical problems initially encountered in the manufacture of synthetic detergent bars ("syndet bars") have now been resolved. As a result of many years of research and development, a product is now available that has been tried and tested under conditions of actual use [6]. It has been shown to meet the dermatologists' requirements and to be suitable for a variety of indications. Equally, it has proved to be cosmetically acceptable. After all, consumers will be persuaded by advertising to buy and consistently use a product only if the product concerned looks nice, smells nice, and lives up to the manufacturer's advertising claims.

References

1. Falbe J (Ed) (1986) Surfactants in Consumer Products. Springer Verlag, Berlin Heidelberg
2. Fiedler HP (1980) In: Korting GW, Dermatologie in Praxis und Klinik Vol 1.7.26. Georg Thieme Verlag, Stuttgart New York
3. Fiedler HP (1986) In: Falbe J (Ed) Surfactants in Consumer Products. Springer Verlag, Berlin Heidelberg
4. Götte E (1960) Fette, Seifen, Anstrichmittel 62: 789
5. Goldemberg RL (1965) J Soc Cosm Chem 16: 317
6. Kiel J (1988) Therapiewoche 38: 3374
7. Lindner K (1964) Tenside – Textilhilfsmittel – Waschrohstoffe. Wissenschaftliche Verlagsgesellschaft Stuttgart Vols I and II 1964, Vol III with contributions from Eicherl E, 1971
8. Raab W (1976) Hautfibel: Medizinische Kosmetik. Fischer-Verlag, Stuttgart
9. Verbeck H (1986) In: Falbe J (Ed) Surfactants in Consumer Products. Springer Verlag, Berlin Heidelberg

The Use of Synthetic Detergent Skin Cleansers – The Community Pharmacist's View

H. Führling

Introduction

As a community pharmacist, I would like to discuss the subject of the use of synthetic cleansers under three headings: the development of this product group, its *present day importance*, and (last, but not least) the pharmacist's *perception* of these products.

As far as the development is concerned, I have been able to follow the events, in my pharmacy, right from the introduction of these cleansers back in 1970.

At that time (1970), *sebamed compact* and *pH5-Eucerin* – to mention but two well-known brand names – were part of the standard range of medicinal products carried by German pharmacies. The term "medicinal products" is being used deliberately, for these products were then treated as "medicines" – i.e. they were dispensed almost exclusively on a doctor's prescription or advice. In our practice, the prescribers were mainly dermatologists and gynaecologists treating patients with sensitive or diseased skins [1]. The standard personal care products were toilet soaps.

Cleanser bars were soon followed by the first liquid cleansers. The medicinal status of the product remained unchanged. One spin-off of the launch of the new product form was an increase in product information.

Data available on *sebamed*, the market leader, showed this cleanser to be non-alkaline, and adjusted to the pH of normal skin (pH 5.5); the cleanser was also known to be insensitive to hard water, i.e. it would not precipitate Ca^{++} and Mg^{++} ions in aqueous solutions, and would, therefore, not form scum.

Prescribability of Synthetic Cleansers

The first major change in the status of synthetic cleansers – if I may call it that – occurred in the mid-"70"s, when the Health Funds (the insurance companies financing health care in Germany) imposed drastic prescribing restrictions for synthetic cleansers.

Patients would now come to the pharmacy with a doctor's *recommendation* rather than a prescription for synthetic cleansers.

However, at the same time, synthetic cleansers were getting better known, and the effects of advertising and recommendation were being supplemented by "word of mouth" publicity along the lines of "My doctor told me …"

For the pharmacist, counselling and the offer of a suitable product range became important functions. Equally, the price of the cleansers was becoming a significant factor, since these products were available from non-pharmacy outlets as well.

These were difficult times, involving much *rethinking and relearning*, as the cleansers ceased to be medicinal or quasi-medicinal articles and were becoming ordinary consumer products. However, pharmacists managed to cope, since the loss of product status was, to some extent, compensated for by the much wider use of the cleansers.

However, as is often the case when sales of a given product increase, there were also more complaints – in the case of synthetic cleansers, customers were reporting excessive defatting and drying of the skin.

Some manufacturers found (or still find) themselves in a dilemma: on the one hand, dermatologists want a sufficiently defatting cleanser to provide adequate treatment of certain disorders [1]; on the other hand, there are many patients with dry skin who tend to use the cleansers *excessively*, thereby producing untoward effects.

One way of remedying the problem is, of course, good user information, stressing the need for following the *instructions* for the use of the cleanser (e.g. to use no more than a large drop of a liquid formulation lathered with water, for the cleansing of the face or other exposed skin areas). Today, a wide range of synthetic cleansers is available in pharmacies. A number of manufacturers offer cleanser bars, liquid cleansers, shampoos, shower preparations, foam baths, and even baby care products, to suit all requirements.

Synthetic cleansers have become established and important articles in the "parapharmaceutical" range of products.

Conclusion

Let us, finally, take a look at the type of client seen by pharmacists today. There are, of course, patients with skin complaints, who have been advised to use synthetic cleansers in the treatment of their disorders. In addition, however, there is a growing number of *healthy users* – young people, or groups of individuals, who feel that their skin is suffering from increased environmental, occupational, or athletic stress.

I believe that this is a promising trend, which, in years to come, should ensure a healthy development of synthetic cleansers among the overall range of skin cleansing products carried by the pharmacy.

References

1. Braun-Falco O, Heilgemeir GP (1981) Syndets zur Reinigung gesunder und erkrankter Haut. Ther Gegenw 120: 1028–1045

The Use of Synthetic Detergent Skin Cleansers – The General Practitioner's View

B. König

Introduction

Far from being just a body cover, human skin is a highly sensitive interface between the individual and his environment.

The skin figures in a variety of idiomatic phrases which show the emotional connotations and associations of the "integument":

Somebody may be described as "thick-skinned" or "thin-skinned"; an actor will try to get "into the skin" of the part he is to play; one may escape by "the skin of one's teeth"; jump "out of one's skin" with fright; or get "under somebody's skin".

While other languages may be richer in skin idioms, there are enough phrases to indicate the way in which, in English, too, the skin is perceived as an organ of sense as well as sensitivity.

When the skin is diseased, the sufferer will feel less attractive, his body image will be compromised, there will be fears of disfigurement and social rejection.

Reactive depression and even suicide attempts have been reported in very severe cases of psoriasis or acne.

Healthy, attractive skin is a source of subjective well-being, of acceptance by, and full functioning in, human society.

For all these reasons, skin care is a must.

The first essential in skin care is proper cleansing of the skin – something that is becoming increasingly important in this day and age, as a result of the relentless increase in environmental factors that stress and irritate the skin.

We are witnessing a considerable rise in the incidence of occupational skin disorders, which have come to account for more than one third of all the occupational diseases reported.

However, skin cleansing in itself – however well meant – can be a source of irritation. Using the wrong kind of cleansing material, washing too often or with too strong an agent can do more harm than good.

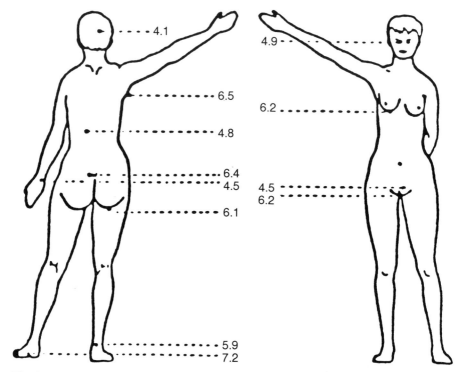

Fig. 1. pH of different skin areas (modified from [3])

pH of Different Skin Areas

Back in 1928–29, Marchionini and Schade discovered that the entire skin is surrounded by an "acid mantle" of regionally different pH; and even earlier, Heuss, Sharlit and Scheer had suggested that this might be so, on the evidence of measurements at various sites.

Subsequent pH measurements in different skin areas essentially provided confirmation of what researchers had found at the start of this century (cf. Fig. 1; [2, 3]).

Protective Function of the Acid Mantle

The maintenance of the acid mantle, or its restoration following cleansing, is of critical importance for the integrity of the skin surface's protective function, especially the defence against microbial attack [1].

Whereas old-fashioned soaps (which are alkali salts of fatty acids) produce alkaline solutions that damage the acid mantle and delay its regeneration, even cleansers of neutral pH are non-physiological.

Acidic synthetic cleansers are much more suitable, since they do not affect the acid mantle to quite the same degree, and permit a more rapid restoration of the mantle after any initial pH displacement caused by washing.

General practitioners, who care for male and female patients of all ages, have come to recommend synthetic skin cleansers in many of the cases seen in day-to-day practice.

Thus, synthetic cleansers, which do not involve occlusion, are superior to the (still widely used) "baby oils" in the care of sensitive baby skin, which takes some weeks to develop its acid mantle, and in the treatment of napkin rash and Candida dermatitis.

While individuals with normal skins will undoubtedly not be harmed by soap, patients with dry skin, ichthyiosis, or endogenous eczema can suffer severe skin irritation when soap is used for cleansing. Synthetic cleansers, with emollients in their formula, do not harbour this risk.

In many skin diseases, the pH is, on average, more alkaline. In such cases, the specific treatment of the disorder can be usefully complemented by washing with acidic synthetic cleansers.

In the management of seborrhoeic disorders (seborrhoea, acne vulgaris, seborrhoeic dermatitis, and rosacea), as well as of candidal paronychias, pityriasis versicolor, erythrasma, miliaria rubra, pompholyx, intertrigo and intertriginous eczema, good use can be made of the drying effect of synthetic cleansers.

Although, to date, no evidence has been provided to show that the acid mantle protects against fungal skin diseases, the regular use of acidic synthetic cleansers will render the habitat less favourable for fungi and produce marked clinical improvement.

Synthetic detergent cleansers also inhibit sweat production, and can therefore be used in all conditions that involve hyperhidrosis. Athletes, who tend to sweat much, often suffer from trichobacteriosis axillaris, as a result of the colonization of axillary hair by coryneform agents, with dense colonies along the hair shafts, and yellow, red, or black discoloration of the sweat, depending on the particular organisms involved.

In bromhidrosis – the production of foul-smelling axillary sweat as a result of microbial decomposition – acidic synthetic cleansers have also proved useful.

In addition to the above-mentioned indications, synthetic cleansers have been successfully employed in general practice to treat the following list of conditions:

Abscesses
Senile pruritus
Prevention of pressure sores
Diabetic skin lesions
Eczema (all types)
Erysipelas
Furunculosis
Kraurosis vulvae
Pruritus vulvae

Psoriasis
Pyoderma
Dry skin
Chickenpox.

Also, these agents have been found useful as a surgical scrub.

In summary, synthetic detergent skin cleansers have become an important part of the general practitioner's armamentarium.

References

1. Braun-Falco O, Heilgemeir GP (1981) Syndets zur Reinigung gesunder und erkrankter Haut. Ther Gegenw 120: 1028
2. Braun-Falco O, Korting HC (1986) Der normale pH-Wert der menschlichen Haut. Hautarzt 37: 126
3. Verut D (1963) J Swed Med Ass 5: 39

The Use of Synthetic Detergent Skin Cleansers – The Consultant Dermatologist's View

G. P. Heilgemeir

Skin Cleansing with Water and Synthetic Detergents

Nowadays, there are a host of surfactants with different properties available to the manufacturer, who can choose from among them to formulate skin cleansers to meet a variety of specifications. Synthetic detergent cleansers have constituted a major breakthrough in the history of skin cleansing.

Acid vs. Alkali

Unlike soaps, synthetic detergent cleansers can be adjusted to an acidic pH, to permit cleansing without damage to the acid mantle of the skin [19, 31]. Even after repeated washing with an acidic synthetic cleanser, no displacement in the skin surface pH was observed [26].

Drying and Defatting

Like water and soap, though in different degrees, synthetic cleansers can affect the water-lipid surface film of the skin [7, 18]. Defatting is largely dependent on the temperature of the washing solution, the concentration of the synthetic cleanser, the time of exposure to the solution, and the skin type of the user. It has also been found that the washing solution can increase the permeability of the skin, making it easier for foreign substances to penetrate [3, 39].

Penetration will be controlled by the time of exposure, and by the chemical nature and concentration of the synthetic detergent in the solution [32]. Also, contact with the washing solution will upset the autoselective ion exchange capacity of the skin, the result being that, depending on the duration and intensity of subsequent rinsing, the surfactants in the solution may be adsorbed to the skin surface as a monomolecular layer that may not be fully rinsable [7]. This surface film makes the skin more wettable, and, being usually hygroscopic, will encourage evaporation from the stratum corneum, and, hence, drying of the skin. The greater the adsorption of the surfactant film, the more pronounced the roughness effect will be. One theory that has been suggested to account for this phenomenon is the formation of complexes between proteins and surfactants, especially anionic ones [7].

Surfactants differ in their penetration, defatting and surface substance leaching properties, and will, therefore produce different degrees of drying and roughness [7, 20]. Also, the drying of the skin is a function of climatic factors [25, 38]. Thus, it is common knowledge that skin tends to be drier in winter than in summer. The skin damage observed after repeated and prolonged exposure to synthetic detergents is chiefly due to insufficient rinsing after use.

Skin irritation and skin defatting by surfactants can be compensated for by the addition to the synthetic detergent of such substances as phospholipids, liposomes, polyols, betaines, sodium lauryl sarcosinate, oatmeal extracts, soya proteins, and sodium salts of higher ethoxylated lauryl sulphates [7].

It has been shown that skin compatibility can be improved also by modifying the chemical structure of the agents involved, to produce a substance of equal or even better cleansing and defatting properties [10]. Superfatting agents can be added to synthetic cleanser formulations, to be deposited on the skin during washing [9, 10, 12].

Ion and Protein Precipitation

Unlike soaps, synthetic detergents do not precipitate magnesium and calcium; they are not hardness sensitive; they produce an immediate detersive effect; and a little goes a long way [19]. One practical benefit is the absence of scum ("bath-tub ring").

Skin irritation by synthetic detergents is thought to be at least partly due to the liberation of SH groups, resulting in the denaturation of keratin [7, 35]. However, no general conclusions can be drawn as to the irritancy of synthetic cleansers, since there are so many different surfactants in the various preparations. Even if taken orally, anionic and nonionic surfactants have little toxicity, while cationic surfactants are only moderately toxic [35].

Antimicrobial Activity

Special additives with different effects (e. g. bacteriostatic and, thus, deodorant) can be incorporated into the formula in order to enlarge the cleanser's spectrum of activity [11, 21, 22]. However, certain surfactants – above all cationic ones – are inherently antimicrobial [34]. The antimicrobial effect of surfactants is produced in various ways. On the one hand, true antimicrobial action has been shown in vitro [24, 27, 28, 29, 40]; on the other hand, the relative drying of the skin by surfactants will affect the growth of micro-organisms.

Also, the washing procedure itself has an effect on the skin flora. Washing is a complex process, as studies of shower baths have shown [14]. Among the factors involved there is the arrangement of skin bacteria in microcolonies between the squames [16, 36], the distribution of the aerobes over the depth of the stratum corneum [1, 30], the microbe dispersing properties of surfactants [6, 16, 36], and the shedding produced by the mechanical action of a jet of water [2, 5, 37].

Contact Allergy

Overall, allergic responses to synthetic cleansers are rare [7, 13]. Skin irritation following the use of synthetic cleansers is most likely to be cumulative irritant in nature, usually as result of improper use or application to an over-sensitive skin.

Antiperspirant Effect

Drying is also promoted by inhibition of perspiration. Under experimental conditions, a 1% sodium lauryl sulphate solution was found to produce an inhibition of sweat production by 25–75% [17].

Use of Synthetic Cleansers in the Treatment of Skin Disorders

In many skin disorders, soap will produce no ill effects. However, it should be obvious from the information given above that, in some skin conditions, healing may be delayed, and severe flare-ups or relapses produced, if the wrong kind of cleanser is applied. Since, however, even diseased skin has to be cleaned, synthetic detergent cleansers are a welcome alternative to soap. These cleansers provide a benefit that goes beyond the mere removal of dirt and grime: Cleanser properties other than detergency can be used in suitable cases to moderate and, indeed, to modify the particular skin condition [4].

Non-alkalinity

Acidic synthetic cleansers have been found particularly useful for individuals who are occupationally exposed to alkaline agents [33, 41]. Synthetic cleansers also have the advantage of not precipitating calcium and magnesium ions. Hence, they can be safely recommended to eczema patients, who, in the past, had to subject themselves to unpopular ("dirty") soap avoidance regimens or risk delayed clearing of their condition. The use of synthetic cleansers has also been found to result in a sparing of anti-eczema medications such as steroids.

Drying and Defatting

Individuals with dry, ichthyotic skins, and those who have to do wet work (housewives) should use emollients or moisturizers if synthetic cleansers are to be used on a long-term basis [33]. However, there are skin conditions where deliberate use may be made of the drying action of these cleansers. Chief among these conditions are seborrhoeic disorders such as seborrhoea, seborrhoeic dermatitis, acne vulgaris, and rosacea. Equally, these cleansers are indicated whenever a skin area is to be "dried out" as part of the management strategy. Thus, the adjuvant use of synthetic cleansers has been found beneficial in candidal paronychias, trichomycosis axillaris, pityriasis versicolor, erythrasma, pompholyx, and miliaria rubra [31]. Also, the cleansers have improved the treatment of intertriginous conditions such as intertrigo, intertriginous eczema, and intertriginous Candida infections, especially in obese subjects, where drying is usually a desirable effect to support the treatment in general.

Protein Precipitation

Synthetic cleansers cause protein denaturation and thus are mildly astringent, a fact that suggests their usefulness in eczema, intertrigo, and conditions involving skin surface loss (cracks, scratches) [4].

Antimicrobial Activity, and Build-up of the Acid Mantle

The use of surfactants is followed by a drop in skin surface pH. This can be put to good use in pyoderma, impetiginized eczema, and, especially, in furunculosis, since the maintenance of the acid mantle permitted by the use of synthetic cleansers will have an adjuvant treatment effect. Also, some synthetic cleansers have antibacterial properties [24]. This is why bromhidrosis (the result of increased bacterial decomposition of sweat) is one of the chief indications for the use of synthetic cleansers [19, 31]. In fungal infections, especially athlete's foot, intertrigo, and tinea cruris, synthetic cleansers have come to be used as disease-specific agents, since they will not only improve the background conditions by their drying action [33] but have also been shown to have antifungal activity [24, 27, 28, 29, 40].

In sports medicine, synthetic cleansers are much appreciated for the frequent washing required by athletes. Since athletes tend to sweat a lot, suffer mechanical skin stress, and often wear occlusive clothing or footwear, they are particularly at risk for bacterial and fungal infections [15].

Some synthetic cleansers have been shown in studies to possess antibacterial and fungistatic activities. These properties can be used for the prevention, by regular washing with these agents, of intertriginous skin conditions and of bacterial and fungal infections [24].

Side Effects

In our experience, synthetic detergent cleansers have been very beneficial, provided they are used physiologically and in suitably selected patients. Irritation has not been a problem, and is only seen if the washing solution used is too strong or too hot, washing is too prolonged, or if the skin is over-sensitive.

Contact allergies are extremely rare and tend to occur only if the detergent contains non-surfactant substances such as disinfectants, formaldehyde, etc. Skin irritation suggests over-intensive use of the cleanser, or over-sensitive skin. Patients with dry skin or atopic dermatitis should be advised to use emollients [4].

In summary, synthetic detergent cleansers are more than just skin cleaning agents. They have become an established management principle in dermatology. It is, therefore, difficult to see why, in the official regulations, they should be deprived of their medicine status and relegated to the rank of mere toiletries.

References

1. Beetz HM (1971) Zur Tiefenverteilung der Hautbakterien im Stratum corneum. Arch Dermatol Forsch 244: 76
2. Bethune DW, Blowers R, Parker M, Pak EA (1965) Dispersal of Staphylococcus aureus by patients and surgical staff. Lancet 2: 458
3. Blank IH, Gould J (1961) Penetration of anionic surfactants into skin. J Invest Dermatol 37: 485
4. Braun-Falco O, Heilgemeir GP (1981) Syndets zur Reinigung gesunder und erkrankter Haut. Ther Gegenw 11: 1028
5. Colaton EJ, Van der Mark JS, Van Toorn MJ (1968) Effect of shower bathing on dispersal of recently acquired transient skin flora. Lancet 1: 865
6. Döll W (1961) Bedeutung und Anwendung grenzflächenaktiver Verbindungen in der Bakteriologie. Fette, Seifen, Anstrichmittel 63: 1071
7. Fiedler HP (1980) Reinigung und Pflege der Haut. In: Korting GW (ed): Dermatologie in Praxis und Klinik. Vol 1. Thieme Verlag, Stuttgart New York
8. Götte E (1963) Grenzflächenaktive Substanzen in ihrer Beziehung zur menschlichen Haut: Aesthet Med 5: 146
9. Gloor M, Falk W, Friedrich HC (1965) Über den Einfluß der Badezusatz-Konzentration und der Badewassertemperatur auf den rückfettenden Effekt von Ölbadezusätzen. Hautarzt 26: 589
10. Gloor M, Falk W, Friedrich HC (1975) Vergleichende Untersuchungen zur Wirkung verschiedener Ölbadezusätze. Z Hautkr 50: 429
11. Gloor M, Ohrmann R (1975) Zur Therapie der Sebostase mit Ölbadezusätzen. Akt Dermatol 1: 273
12. Gloor M, Tretow CW, Friedrich HC (1974) Über die Beeinflussung der Hautoberflächenlipide durch Körperreinigungsmittel. Dermatol Monatsschr 160: 291
13. Grimmer H, Jung E, Klaschka F, Krüger HG, Schwarz T, Wagner W (1975) Spezielle Netzmittelkombinationen als physikalisch-therapeutisches Behandlungsprinzip bei Erkrankungen des behaarten Kopfes. Zeitschr Hautkr 50: 253
14. Hartmann AA (1980) Duschbaden und sein Einfluß auf die aerobe Residentflora der menschlichen Haut. Arch Dermatol Res 267: 161
15. Heilgemeir GP (1984) Häufig waschen ja – aber nicht mit Seife. Ärztl Prax 5: 77–79

16. Holt RJ (1971) Aerobic bacterial counts on human skin after bathing. J Med Microbiol 4: 391
17. Hölzle E, Kligman AM (1979) Selective damage of the acrosyringium by watersoluble irritants. J Invest Dermatol 72: 276
18. Ivanov VV (1976) Experimentelles Studium der Wirkung von einigen Seifen auf die Haut. Vestn Derm Vener 3: 57
19. Keining E (196) Die Hautpflege mit synthetischen Detergentien. Ärztl Prax 103: 5788
20. Kirk JF (1966) Effect of hand washing on skin lipid removal. Acta Derm Venereol Suppl 57: 24
21. Kürner H (1975) Therapeutischer Erfahrungsbericht mit der Avena-Reihe. Zschr Haut Geschlkr 50: 631
22. Leyh F (1973) Schutz, Pflege und Reinigung der Haut in Abhängigkeit vom Arbeitsplatz. Hautarzt 24: 415
23. Marchionini A, Schade H (1928) Der Säuremantel der Haut (nach Gaskettenmessungen). Klin Wochenschr 7: 12
24. Marghescu S (1970) Die Intertrigo, ihre Prophylaxe und Behandlung. Ther Gegenw 6: 813
25. Middleton JD (1969) The effect of temperature on extensibility of isolated stratum corneum and its relation to skin chapping. Brit J Dermatol 81: 717
26. Möhn R, Schimpf A (1973) Zum Waschverbot bei Ekzemkrankheiten. Ther Gegenw 1: 98
27. Qadripur A, Gründer K (1974) Untersuchungen über die antimycetische Wirksamkeit waschaktiver Substanzen. Hautarzt 25: 618
28. Rieth H (1976) Dekontamination mit synthetischen Detergentien. Pilzsprechstunde 2: 50
29. Rieth H, Abou-Gabel M (1969) Nachweis der pilzhemmenden Wirkung von Stephalen-Waschgel. Mykosen 12: 511
30. Röckl H, Müller E (1959) Beitrag zur Lokalisation der Mikroben der Haut. Arch klin exper Dermatol 209: 13
31. Roth WG (1969) Bedeutung der Syndets für die gesunde und pathologisch veränderte Haut. Ärztl Prax 20: 1193
32. Scala J, Osker DE, Reller HH (1968) The percutaneous absorption of ionic surfactants. J Invest Dermatol 50: 371
33. Schneider W (1961) Seifen und Syndets. Aesthet Med 10: 304
34. Schneider W, Tronnier H, Wagner H (1962) Reinigung und Pflege der Haut im Beruf unter besonderer Berücksichtigung der experimentellen und praktischen Prüfverfahren. In: Gottron HA Schönfeld W (eds): Dermatologie und Venereologie Vol 1, Part 2. Thieme-Verlag, Stuttgart New York
35. Smeenk G (1969) The influence of detergents on the skin. Arch klin exper Dermatol 235: 180
36. Sommerville DA, Noble CW (1973) Microcolony size of microbes on human skin. J Med Microbiol 6: 323
37. Speers RJ, Bernard H, Grady FO, Shooter (1965) Increased dispersal of skin bacteria into the air after shower-bath. Lancet 1: 478
38. Spencer S, Linamen CE, Akers WA, Jones HE (1975) Temperature dependence of water content of stratum corneum. Brit J Dermatol 93: 159
39. Stüpel H, Szakall A (1957) Die Wirkung von Waschmitteln auf die Haut. Hüthig-Verlag, Heidelberg
40. Thianprasit M (1963) Zur Frage des antimykotischen Effekts von Seifen und Syndets. Dermatol Wochenschr 147: 649
41. Weber G (1979) Hautreinigung und Hautpflege im Berufsleben. Arbeitsmedizin, Sozialmedizin, Präventivmedizin 7: 167